Medical Devices

Related titles

Standardisation in Cell and Tissue Engineering
(ISBN: 978-0-85709-419-3)

Biocompatibility and Performance of Medical Devices
(ISBN: 978-0-85709-070-6)

Regulatory Affairs for Biomedical Devices
(ISBN: 978-0-85709-542-8)

Woodhead Publishing Series in Biomaterials: Number 103

Medical Devices

Regulations, Standards and Practices

Seeram Ramakrishna
Lingling Tian, Charlene Wang
Susan Liao and Wee Eong Teo

ELSEVIER

AMSTERDAM • BOSTON • CAMBRIDGE • HEIDELBERG
LONDON • NEW YORK • OXFORD • PARIS • SAN DIEGO
SAN FRANCISCO • SINGAPORE • SYDNEY • TOKYO
Woodhead Publishing is an imprint of Elsevier

WP
WOODHEAD
PUBLISHING

Woodhead Publishing is an imprint of Elsevier
80 High Street, Sawston, Cambridge, CB22 3HJ, UK
225 Wyman Street, Waltham, MA 02451, USA
Langford Lane, Kidlington, OX5 1GB, UK

ISBN: 978-0-08-100289-6 (Print)
ISBN: 978-0-08-100291-9 (Online)

British Library Cataloguing in Publication Data
A catalogue record for this book is available from the British Library

Library of Congress Control Number: 2015939559

For information on all Woodhead Publishing publications
visit our website at http://store.elsevier.com/

Printed and bound in the United Kingdom

Contents

List of contributors

Susan Liao Nanyang Technological University, Singapore

Seeram Ramakrishna National University of Singapore, Singapore & Guangdong-Hong Kong-Macau Institute of CNS Regeneration, Jinan University, Guangzhou, PR China

Wee Eong Teo National University of Singapore, Singapore

LingLing Tian National University of Singapore, Singapore & Guangdong-Hong Kong-Macau Institute of CNS Regeneration, Jinan University, Guangzhou, PR China

Charlene Wang National University of Singapore, Singapore

Woodhead Publishing Series in Biomaterials

1 **Sterilisation of tissues using ionising radiations**
Edited by J. F. Kennedy, G. O. Phillips and P. A. Williams
2 **Surfaces and interfaces for biomaterials**
Edited by P. Vadgama
3 **Molecular interfacial phenomena of polymers and biopolymers**
Edited by C. Chen
4 **Biomaterials, artificial organs and tissue engineering**
Edited by L. Hench and J. Jones
5 **Medical modelling**
R. Bibb
6 **Artificial cells, cell engineering and therapy**
Edited by S. Prakash
7 **Biomedical polymers**
Edited by M. Jenkins
8 **Tissue engineering using ceramics and polymers**
Edited by A. R. Boccaccini and J. Gough
9 **Bioceramics and their clinical applications**
Edited by T. Kokubo
10 **Dental biomaterials**
Edited by R. V. Curtis and T. F. Watson
11 **Joint replacement technology**
Edited by P. A. Revell
12 **Natural-based polymers for biomedical applications**
Edited by R. L. Reiss et al
13 **Degradation rate of bioresorbable materials**
Edited by F. J. Buchanan
14 **Orthopaedic bone cements**
Edited by S. Deb
15 **Shape memory alloys for biomedical applications**
Edited by T. Yoneyama and S.Miyazaki
16 **Cellular response to biomaterials**
Edited by L. Di Silvio
17 **Biomaterials for treating skin loss**
Edited by D. P. Orgill and C. Blanco
18 **Biomaterials and tissue engineering in urology**
Edited by J.Denstedt and A. Atala
19 **Materials science for dentistry**
B. W. Darvell
20 **Bone repair biomaterials**
Edited by J. A. Planell, S. M. Best, D. Lacroix and A. Merolli

21 **Biomedical composites**
Edited by L. Ambrosio
22 **Drug–device combination products**
Edited by A. Lewis
23 **Biomaterials and regenerative medicine in ophthalmology**
Edited by T. V. Chirila
24 **Regenerative medicine and biomaterials for the repair of connective tissues**
Edited by C. Archer and J. Ralphs
25 **Metals for biomedical devices**
Edited by M. Ninomi
26 **Biointegration of medical implant materials: Science and design**
Edited by C. P. Sharma
27 **Biomaterials and devices for the circulatory system**
Edited by T. Gourlay and R. Black
28 **Surface modification of biomaterials: Methods analysis and applications**
Edited by R. Williams
29 **Biomaterials for artificial organs**
Edited by M. Lysaght and T. Webster
30 **Injectable biomaterials: Science and applications**
Edited by B. Vernon
31 **Biomedical hydrogels: Biochemistry, manufacture and medical applications**
Edited by S. Rimmer
32 **Preprosthetic and maxillofacial surgery: Biomaterials, bone grafting and tissue engineering**
Edited by J. Ferri and E. Hunziker
33 **Bioactive materials in medicine: Design and applications**
Edited by X. Zhao, J. M. Courtney and H. Qian
34 **Advanced wound repair therapies**
Edited by D. Farrar
35 **Electrospinning for tissue regeneration**
Edited by L. Bosworth and S. Downes
36 **Bioactive glasses: Materials, properties and applications**
Edited by H. O. Ylänen
37 **Coatings for biomedical applications**
Edited by M. Driver
38 **Progenitor and stem cell technologies and therapies**
Edited by A. Atala
39 **Biomaterials for spinal surgery**
Edited by L. Ambrosio and E. Tanner
40 **Minimized cardiopulmonary bypass techniques and technologies**
Edited by T. Gourlay and S. Gunaydin
41 **Wear of orthopaedic implants and artificial joints**
Edited by S. Affatato
42 **Biomaterials in plastic surgery: Breast implants**
Edited by W. Peters, H. Brandon, K. L. Jerina, C. Wolf and V. L. Young
43 **MEMS for biomedical applications**
Edited by S. Bhansali and A. Vasudev
44 **Durability and reliability of medical polymers**
Edited by M. Jenkins and A. Stamboulis
45 **Biosensors for medical applications**
Edited by S. Higson

46 **Sterilisation of biomaterials and medical devices**
Edited by S. Lerouge and A. Simmons
47 **The hip resurfacing handbook: A practical guide to the use and management of modern hip resurfacings**
Edited by K. De Smet, P. Campbell and C. Van Der Straeten
48 **Developments in tissue engineered and regenerative medicine products**
J. Basu and J. W. Ludlow
49 **Nanomedicine: Technologies and applications**
Edited by T. J. Webster
50 **Biocompatibility and performance of medical devices**
Edited by J-P. Boutrand
51 **Medical robotics: Minimally invasive surgery**
Edited by P. Gomes
52 **Implantable sensor systems for medical applications**
Edited by A. Inmann and D. Hodgins
53 **Non-metallic biomaterials for tooth repair and replacement**
Edited by P. Vallittu
54 **Joining and assembly of medical materials and devices**
Edited by Y. (Norman) Zhou and M. D. Breyen
55 **Diamond-based materials for biomedical applications**
Edited by R.Narayan
56 **Nanomaterials in tissue engineering: Fabrication and applications**
Edited by A. K. Gaharwar, S. Sant, M. J. Hancock and S. A. Hacking
57 **Biomimetic biomaterials: Structure and applications**
Edited by A. J. Ruys
58 **Standardisation in cell and tissue engineering: Methods and protocols**
Edited by V. Salih
59 **Inhaler devices: Fundamentals, design and drug delivery**
Edited by P. Prokopovich
60 **Bio-tribocorrosion in biomaterials and medical implants**
Edited by Y. Yan
61 **Microfluidic devices for biomedical applications**
Edited by X-J. James Li and Y. Zhou
62 **Decontamination in hospitals and healthcare**
Edited by J. T. Walker
63 **Biomedical imaging: Applications and advances**
Edited by P. Morris
64 **Characterization of biomaterials**
Edited by M. Jaffe, W. Hammond, P. Tolias and T. Arinzeh
65 **Biomaterials and medical tribology**
Edited by J. Paolo Davim
66 **Biomaterials for cancer therapeutics: Diagnosis, prevention and therapy**
Edited by K. Park
67 **New functional biomaterials for medicine and healthcare**
E.P. Ivanova, K.Bazaka and R. J. Crawford
68 **Porous silicon for biomedical applications**
Edited by H. A. Santos
69 **A practical approach to spinal trauma**
Edited by H. N. Bajaj and S. Katoch
70 **Rapid prototyping of biomaterials: Principles and applications**
Edited by R.Narayan

71 **Cardiac regeneration and repair Volume 1: Pathology and therapies**
Edited by R-K. Li and R. D. Weisel
72 **Cardiac regeneration and repair Volume 2: Biomaterials and tissue engineering**
Edited by R-K. Li and R. D. Weisel
73 **Semiconducting silicon nanowires for biomedical applications**
Edited by J.L. Coffer
74 **Silk biomaterials for tissue engineering and regenerative medicine**
Edited by S. Kundu
75 **Biomaterials for bone regeneration: Novel techniques and applications**
Edited by P.Dubruel and S. Van Vlierberghe
76 **Biomedical foams for tissue engineering applications**
Edited by P. Netti
77 **Precious metals for biomedical applications**
Edited by N. Baltzer and T. Copponnex
78 **Bone substitute biomaterials**
Edited by K. Mallick
79 **Regulatory affairs for biomaterials and medical devices**
Edited by S. F. Amato and R. Ezzell
80 **Joint replacement technology Second edition**
Edited by P. A. Revell
81 **Computational modelling of biomechanics and biotribology in the musculoskeletal system: Biomaterials and tissues**
Edited by Z. Jin
82 **Biophotonics for medical applications**
Edited by I. Meglinski
83 **Modelling degradation of bioresorbable polymeric medical devices**
Edited by J. Pan
84 **Perspectives in total hip arthroplasty: Advances in biomaterials and their tribological interactions**
S. Affatato
85 **Tissue engineering using ceramics and polymers Second edition**
Edited by A. R. Boccaccini and P. X. Ma
86 **Biomaterials and medical-device associated infections**
Edited by L. Barnes and I. R. Cooper
87 **Surgical techniques in total knee arthroplasty (TKA) and alternative procedures**
Edited by S. Affatato
88 **Lanthanide oxide nanoparticles for molecular imaging and therapeutics**
G. H. Lee
89 **Surface modification of magnesium and its alloys for biomedical applications Volume 1: Biological interactions, mechanical properties and testing**
Edited by T. S. N. Sankara Narayanan, I. S. Park and M. H. Lee
90 **Surface modification of magnesium and its alloys for biomedical applications Volume 2: Modification and coating techniques**
Edited by T. S. N. Sankara Narayanan, I. S. Park and M. H. Lee
91 **Medical modelling: The application of advanced design and rapid prototyping techniques in medicine Second Edition**
Edited by R. Bibb, D. Eggbeer and A. Paterson
92 **Switchable and responsive surfaces and materials for biomedical applications**
Edited by Z. Zhang
93 **Biomedical textiles for orthopaedic and surgical applications: Fundamentals, applications and tissue engineering**
Edited by T. Blair

94 **Surface coating and modification of metallic biomaterials**
Edited by C. Wen

95 **Hydroxyapatite (HAP) for biomedical applications**
Edited by M. Mucalo

96 **Implantable neuroprostheses for restoring function**
Edited by K. Kilgore

97 **Shape memory polymers for biomedical applications**
Edited by L. Yahia

98 **Regenerative engineering of musculoskeletal tissues and interfaces**
Edited by S.P. Nukavarapu, J.W. Freeman and C.T. Laurencin

99 **Advances in cardiac imaging: Techniques and applications**
Edited by K. Nieman, O. Gaemperli, P. Lancellotti and S. Plein

100 **Functional marine biomaterials: Properties and applications**
Edited by Se-Kwon Kim

101 **Shoulder and elbow trauma and its complications: Volume 1: The shoulder**
Edited by R. M. Greiwe

102 **Nanotechnology-enhanced orthopaedic materials: Applications and future trends**
Edited by L. Yang

103 **Medical devices: Regulations, standards and practices**
Edited by Seeram Ramakrishna, Lingling Tian, Charlene Wang, Susan Liao and Wee Eong Teo

Introduction

1

1.1 Medical devices: definitions and types

Definitions of medical devices have been summarized in Table 1.1 [1–4]. Although they are slightly different, main descriptions of medical devices are generally similar. Other than drugs, medical-related instruments, apparatuses, implements, machines, appliances, implants, *in vitro* reagents or calibrators, software, materials or other similarly related articles are considered medical devices.

Examples of medical devices range from something as simple as bandages, medical thermometers, stethoscopes, or disposable gloves to advanced devices such as equipment and/or computers with software that assists in the conducting of medical tests (e.g., MRI, ultrasound, CT), implants, and prostheses; there are approximately 1.5 million different devices. Medical devices vary greatly in complexity and application. Current medical devices can replace almost every part of the human body (Figure 1.1) with partial to full functional support. The development of medical devices witnessed steady growth as increasing innovative factors became involved. For example, contact lenses which have been used widely as vision aid and for aesthetic purposes may have additional functions in the future. Google and Novartis are working on smart contact lenses, thus we foresee eyewear that will be able to monitor blood-sugar levels for diabetics. (Figure 1.2) [5].

The different regulatory authorities in each country recognize different classes of medical devices based on their design complexity, their use characteristics, and their potential safety hazard if misused. Each country defines these categories in different ways. But typically, they are regulated into class I, II (IIa, IIb), and III (or A, B, C, D) based on the risk level to patients, ranging from low risk to high risk (Table 1.2). Higher-risk devices require stricter control by the respective regulatory authorities to ensure their safe use and performance effectiveness. Detailed classifications from various countries will be further described in Chapter 2. The categorization of medical devices was based on the nature of body contact and contact duration for the ISO 10993 biocompatibility test. Table 1.3 [6] lists several examples under this categorization. The categorization will determine what biocompatibility tests should be done before clinical trials; this will be further illustrated in Chapter 6.

The authorities also recognize that some devices are provided in combination with drugs, the regulation of these combination products takes this factor into consideration and the USFDA established the office of combination products in 2002 to regulate these products. Tissue-engineered products are treated as combination products because they are usually comprised of a cellular or tissue component as well as a device component, thus they need to go through separate reviews for each component.

Medical devices. http://dx.doi.org/10.1016/B978-0-08-100289-6.00001-6

Table 1.1 Definition of medical device

Organization	Definition	Type	Resource and issue date	Remarks
US FDA	"An instrument, apparatus, implement, machine, contrivance, implant, *in vitro* reagent, or other similar or related article, including a component part, or accessory which is: • recognized in the official National Formulary, or the United States Pharmacopoeia, or any supplement to them, • intended for use in the diagnosis of disease or other conditions, or in the cure, mitigation, treatment, or prevention of disease, in man or other animals, • or intended to affect the structure or any function of the body of man or other animals, and which does not achieve its primary intended purposes through chemical action within or on the body of man or other animals • and which is not dependent upon being metabolized for the achievement of any of its primary intended purposes" [1].	Class I, II, & III	In section 201(h) by Federal Food, Drugs, and Cosmetic Act (FD&C), 2006 Edition, Supplement 3 current through January 5, 2010.	The definition provides a clear distinction between a medical device and other FDA regulated products such as drugs.
WHO GHTF SGI	any instrument, apparatus, implement, machine, appliance, implant, reagent for *in vitro* use, software, material or other similar or related article, intended by the manufacturer to be used, alone or in combination, for human beings, for one or more of the specific medical purpose(s) of: • diagnosis, prevention, monitoring, treatment or alleviation of disease, • diagnosis, monitoring, treatment, alleviation of or compensation for an injury,		revision of GHTF/SG1/N29:2005, May 16, 2012	Products which may be considered to be medical devices in some jurisdictions but not in others include: disinfection substances, aids for persons with disabilities, devices incorporating animal and/or human tissues,

	• investigation, replacement, modification, or support of the anatomy or of a physiological process.
	• supporting or sustaining life,
	• control of conception,
	  ◦ disinfection of medical devices,
	  ◦ providing information by means of *in vitro* examination of specimens derived from the human body;
	
	and does not achieve its primary intended action by pharmacological,
	immunological or metabolic means, in or on the human body, but which may be assisted in its intended function by such means [2].
				devices for *in vitro* fertilization or assisted reproduction technologies.

EU	Any instrument, apparatus, appliance, software, material or other article, whether used alone or in combination, together with any accessories, including the software intended by its manufacturer to be used specifically for diagnostic and/or therapeutic purposes and necessary for its proper application, intended by the manufacturer to be used for human beings for the purpose of: • diagnosis, prevention, monitoring, treatment, or alleviation of disease • diagnosis, monitoring, treatment, alleviation of, or compensation for an injury or handicap • investigation, replacement, or modification of the anatomy or of a physiological process • control of conception	Class I, IIa, IIb, and III	Directive 2007/47/EC, 5 September 2007	

Continued

Table 1.1 Continued

Organization	Definition	Type	Resource and issue date	Remarks
	This includes devices that do not achieve their principal intended action in or on the human body by pharmacological, immunological, or metabolic means—but may be assisted in their function by such means [3].			
ISO 13485	any instrument, apparatus, implement, machine, appliance, implant, *in vitro* reagent or calibrator, software, material or other similar or related article, intended by the manufacturer to be used, alone or in combination, for human beings for one or more of the specific purpose(s) of • diagnosis, prevention, monitoring, treatment or alleviation of disease, • diagnosis, monitoring, treatment, alleviation of or compensation for an injury. • investigation, replacement, modification, or support of the anatomy or of a physiological process, • supporting or sustaining life, • control of conception, • disinfection of medical devices, • providing information for medical purposes by means of *in vitro* examination of specimens derived from the human body, and which does not achieve its primary intended action in or on the human body by pharmacological, immunological or metabolic means, but which may be assisted in its function by such means [4].		July 2012, it supersedes ISO 13485:2003 Related to Directives 90/385/EEC,93/42/EEC and 98/79/EC. Resource from: Global Harmonization Task Force (GHTF) – Study Group 1 (SG1), Document No. N029R11, dated 2 February, 2002	Most updated version.

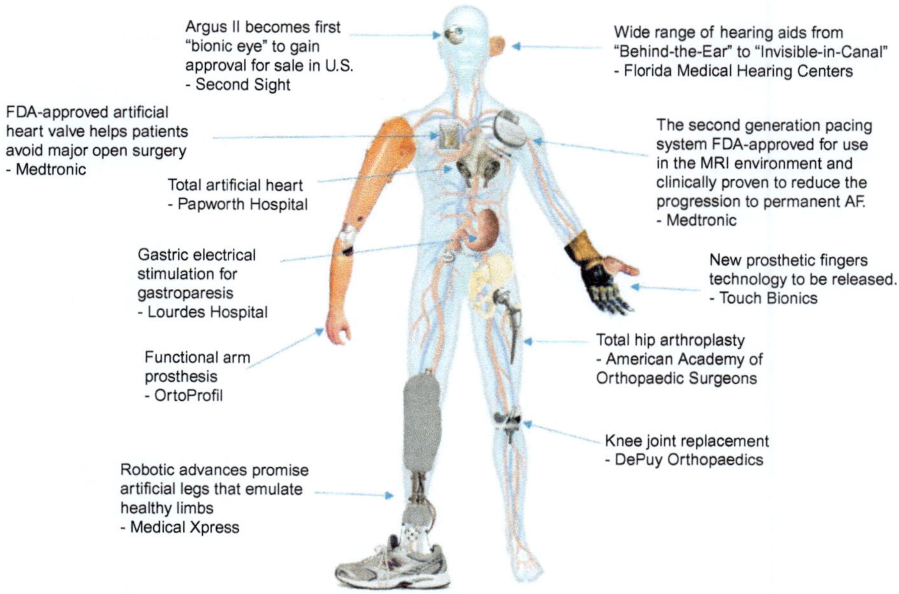

Figure 1.1 Examples of medical devices for the human body.

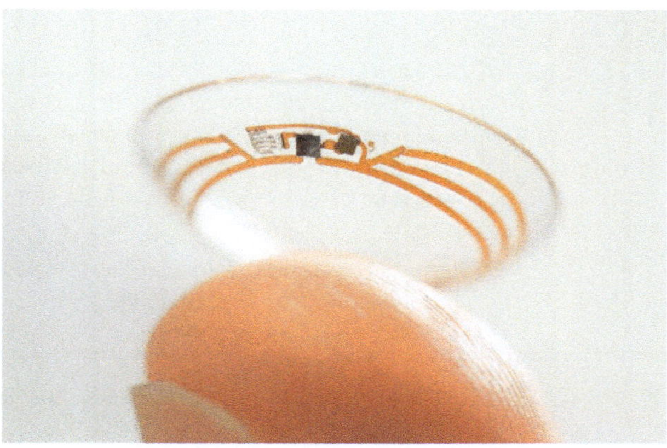

Figure 1.2 An example of smart contact lens [5].

Table 1.2 Examples of medical devices based on Singapore classification [HSA GN-15]

Class	Risk level	Devices examples
A	Low risk	Surgical retractors; tongue depressors
B	Low-moderate risk	Hypodermic needles; suction equipment
C	Moderate-high risk	Lung ventilator; bone fracture fixation plate
D	High risk	Heart valves; implantable defibrillator

The content is accurate as of July 2015, please refer to HSA website for updated information.

Table 1.3 Categorization of medical devices [ISO 10993]

Nature of body contact	Examples
Surface-contacting devices	
Skin	Electrodes, external prostheses, fixation tapes, compression bandages and monitors of various types
Mucosal membranes	Contact lenses, urinary catheters, intravaginal and intra-intestinal devices (stomach tubes, sigmoidoscopies, colonoscopies, gastroscopes), endotracheal tubes, bronchoscopes, some dental prostheses and orthodontic devices
Breached or compromised surfaces	Dressings or healing devices and occlusive patches, for ulcers, burns and granulation tissue
External communicating devices	
Blood path, indirect	Solution administration sets, extension sets, transfer sets and blood administration sets
Tissue/bone/dentin	Laparoscopes, arthroscopes, draining systems, dental cements, dental filling materials and skin staples
Circulating blood	Intravascular catheters, temporary pacemaker electrodes, oxygenators, extracorporal oxygenator tubing and accessories, dialysers, dialysis tubing and accessories, haemoadsorbents and immunoadsorbents
Implant devices	
Tissue/bone	Pacemakers, drug supply devices, neuromuscular sensors and simulators, replacement tendons, breast implants, artificial larynxes, subperiosteal implants, ligation clips and intra-uterine devices; orthopaedic pins, plates, replacement joints, bone prostheses, bone cements and intra-osseous devices
Blood	Pacemaker electrodes, artificial arteriovenous fistulae, heart valves, vascular grafts, internal drug-delivery catheters and ventricular assist devices

1.2 Market trend

The global medical device market reached approximately $363.8 billion in 2013 [7] with annual average growth of the global market around 18.41% [8] from 2010 to 2020. Figure 1.3 reflects the global market share, which mainly consisted of North America, Europe, and Asia-Pacific, the rest of the world only makes up 6% of the market share. The top 10 medical device markets by sales revenue in 2012 are United States (36.3%), Japan (9.9%), Germany (7.0%), China (4.3%), France (4.1%), UK (3.0%), Italy (2.6%), Russia (2.1%), Canada (2.1%), and Brazil (1.6) [9]. In recent

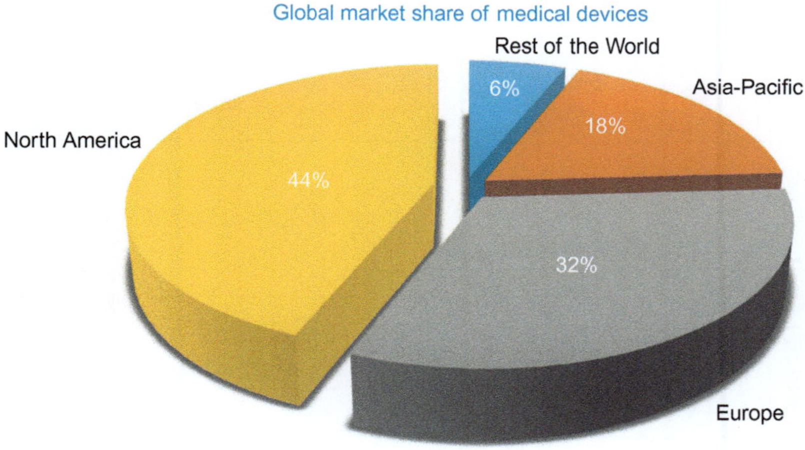

Figure 1.3 Global market share of medical devices.

years, the four BRIC markets (Brazil, Russia, India, and China) have rapidly grown to a total market of US$26.2 billion in 2012. While Chinese per capita spending remains low in absolute terms at US$10.5, the Chinese market was the fourth largest market in the world during 2012 and it is forecasted to become the second largest by 2017 [10]. The top 20 companies in the medical device market are listed in Table 1.4 [7], the top 3 companies were Johnson & Johnson (J&J), Siemens, and Medtronic, respectively, in 2013. These top companies invested 8.1% in R&D as indicated in Figure 1.4. Orthopedics and cardiovascular are the two largest medical device market areas in the United States. J&J mainly dominates the slow-growing orthopedics market with sales of US$8.9 billion and a 26.5% market share in 2013 (Figure 1.5) while Medtronic was predicted to maintain in the top spot for cardiology from 2013 to 2020 with sales of US $8.8 billion and a 22.2% market share in 2013 (Figure 1.6) [7]. The design of medical devices has developed into a major segment of the field of biomedical engineering, which is multidisciplinary, related to biology, medicine, materials and engineering, etc. Most universities have already established bioengineering departments to educate students in this field. Those students join biomedical companies to contribute to the development of the medical device industry upon graduation.

The driving forces behind the development of the medical device market are: 1) longer life span with a growing aging population, 2) higher quality of life and changing life styles; 3) public awareness, all stakeholders are sharing the awareness and responsibility (Figure 1.7). In almost every country, the population aged 60 years and above is growing faster than any other age group, as a result of both longer life expectancy and declining birth rates. For example, the life expectancy in Singapore has increased from 75 to 83 years old from 1990 to 2012 [11]. Seventy years was the average life expectancy rate of the global population in 2012 [12]. With the development of positive medical devices, patients are diagnosed at early stages and receive timely treatments, significantly improving their quality of life both in the hospital and at home even with permanent injury as compared to before.

Table 1.4 WW Medtech Sales: top 20 companies and total market (2013/2020) [7]

Company	Country	WW Medtech Sales ($bn)			WW Market Share			Rank
		2013	2020	%CAGR 13-20	2013 (%)	2020 (%)	Chg. (+/−)	Chg. (+/−)
Johnson & Johnson	USA	28.5	32.8	+2.0	7.8	6.4	−1.4pp	–
Siemens	Germany	17.9	24.0	+4.3	4.9	4.7	−0.2pp	–
Medtronic	USA	17.0	22.1	+3.8	4.7	4.3	−0.4pp	–
Roche	Switzerland	11.3	15.3	+4.4	3.1	3.0	−0.1pp	–
Covidien	USA	10.2	13.8	+4.4	2.8	2.7	−0.1pp	–
Abbott Laboratories	USA	9.9	13.7	+4.8	2.7	2.7	−0.0pp	–
Stryker	USA	9.0	13.1	+5.4	2.5	2.5	+0.1pp	+2
General Electric	USA	9.8	12.0	+3.0	2.7	2.3	−0.3pp	−1
Philips	The Netherlands	9.4	11.6	+3.0	2.6	2.3	−0.3pp	−1
Essilor International	France	6.0	10.4	+8.2	1.6	2.0	+0.4pp	+5
Danaher	USA	7.0	9.6	+4.7	1.9	1.9	−0.0pp	–
Becton Dickinson	USA	7.0	9.4	+4.4	1.9	1.8	−0.1pp	+1
Baxter International	USA	5.8	9.3	+7.0	1.6	1.8	+0.2pp	+3
Boston Scientific	USA	7.1	9.3	+3.8	2.0	1.8	−0.2pp	−4
B. Braun Melsungen	Germany	6.9	9.2	+4.3	1.9	1.8	−0.1pp	−1
Novartis	Switzerland	7.0	9.0	+3.8	1.9	1.8	−0.2pp	−4
Olympus	Japan	4.9	8.0	+7.2	1.4	1.6	+0.2pp	+2
St. Jude Medical	USA	5.5	7.5	+4.6	1.5	1.5	−0.0pp	−1
3M	USA	5.1	7.1	+4.8	1.4	1.4	−0.0pp	−1
Smith & Nephew	United Kingdom	4.4	6.4	+5.7	1.2	1.2	+0.1pp	+2
Total top 20		189.6	253.5	+4.2	52.1	49.4	−2.7pp	
Other		174.2	260.0	+5.9	47.9	50.6	+2.7pp	
Total		363.8	513.5	+5.0	100.0	100.0		

Note: Analysis based on the top 200 medtech companies. Sales in 2013 based on company reported data. Sales forecasts to 2020 based on consensus of leading equity.
Source: EvaluateMedTech World Preview 2014, Outlook to 2020. Copyright © 2015 Evaluate Ltd. All rights reserved. www.evaluate.com.

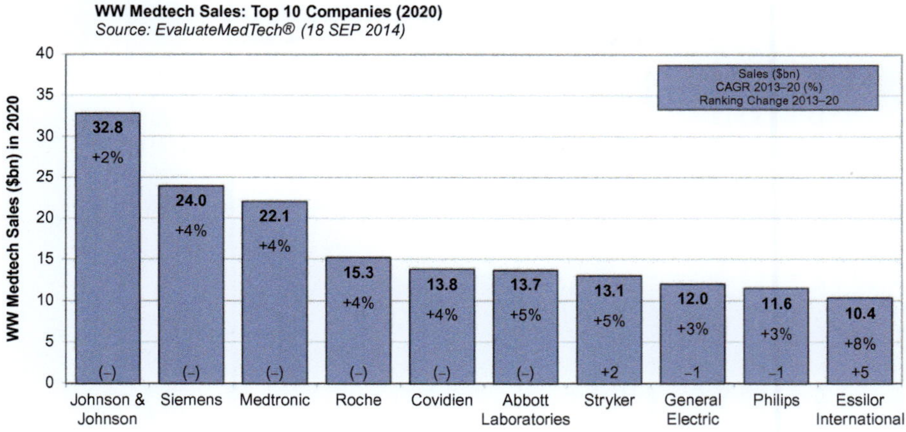

Figure 1.4 Top 10 companies in medical device sales [7].
EvaluateMedTech World Preview 2014, Outlook to 2020. Copyright © 2015 Evaluate Ltd. All rights reserved. www.evaluate.com.

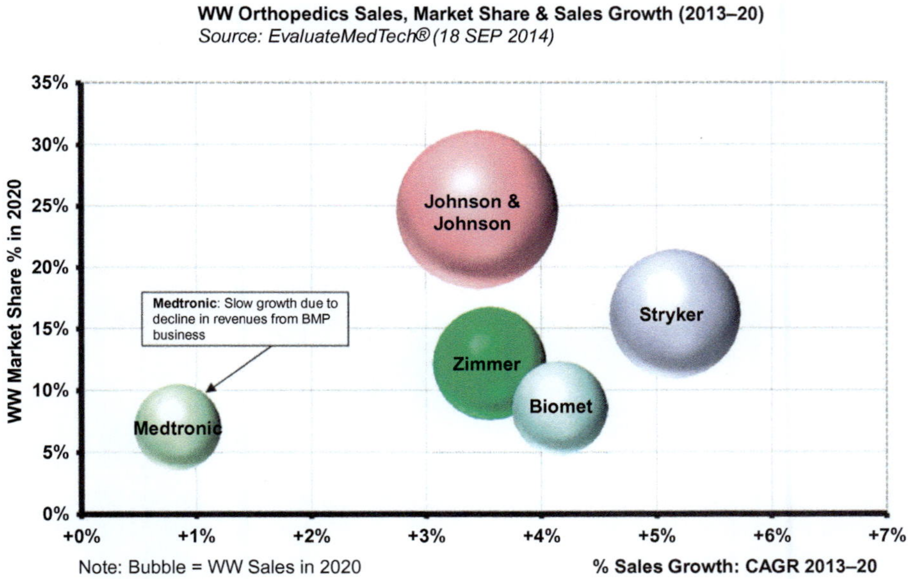

Figure 1.5 Top five companies in orthopedics medical device sales [7].
EvaluateMedTech World Preview 2014, Outlook to 2020. Copyright © 2015 Evaluate Ltd. All rights reserved. www.evaluate.com.

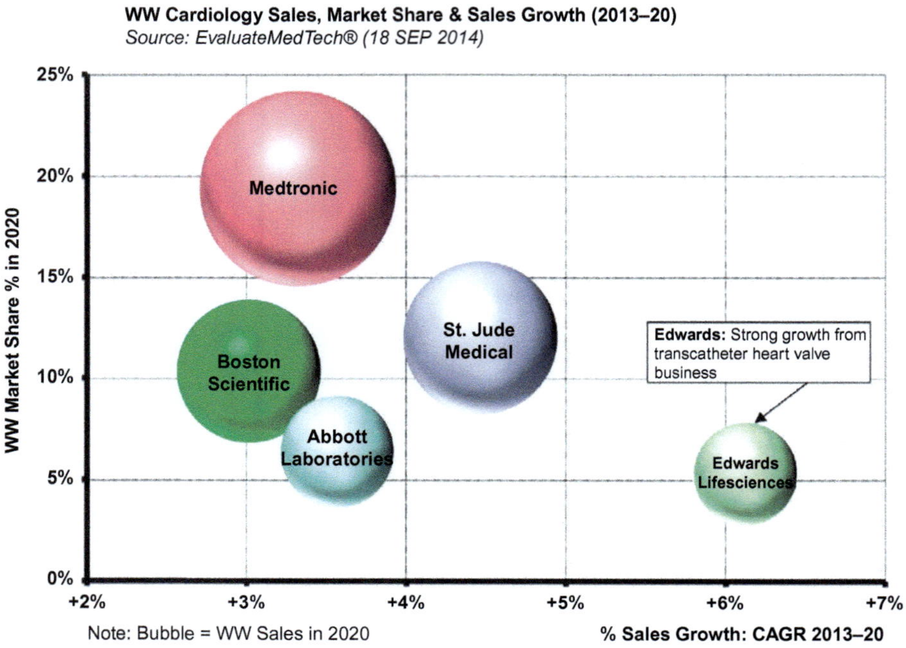

Figure 1.6 Top 5 companies in cardiology medical device sales [7].
EvaluateMedTech World Preview 2014, Outlook to 2020. www.evaluate.com.

Figure 1.7 Drivers of growth for medical devices.

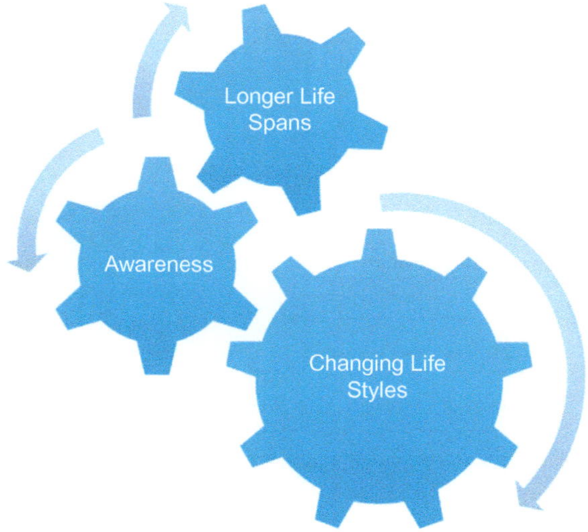

1.3 Safety issues

Although the purpose of medical devices is to help solve health problems, not all medical devices are confirmed to be safe for use at the beginning of a design stage. In other words, the benefits of the new device must outweigh the risks brought about by the device to the patient; this is the evaluation standard used before marketing a device. Several adverse event report systems have been established recently to monitor those marketed devices and to keep the relevant manufacturer, doctor, patient, and the public informed. The medical device researchers and developers can learn from the history of medical device safety issues.

Safe devices must be constructed from safe raw materials; the composition of the materials that make up the device should be clear as any potential leaching materials would present a hazard. We often see the bisphenol A (BPA)-free label on water containers. Both BPA and phthalates are suspected to be endocrine disruptors. Endocrine disruptors are chemicals that may interfere with the production or activity of hormones in the human endocrine system. Phthalate plasticizers have been used to fabricate disposable medical devices for over 60 years. Disposable device refers to one time use only, which is very crucial for infection control and brings tremendous convenience to medical treatment. However, toxicity reports on chemical additives in polyvinylchloride (PVC) early in 1960s were observed. Particularly di-2-ethylbenzyl phthalate (DEHP) at low concentration causes liver damage and at a high level in diet it causes liver cancer in rodents [13]. Leaching of DEHP from PVC blood bags & tubes into blood and blood products stored in such bags greatly exposed the dialysis patients, hemophiliacs, or people who received blood transfusions to DEHP [13]. DEHP is listed as "reasonably anticipated to be a human carcinogen" in the twelfth report on carcinogens published by the National Toxicology Program [14] although the effects of phthalates on human health is not fully known yet. The National Toxicology Program also concluded that high levels of one phthalate-DEPH may adversely affect human reproduction or development [14]. Thus, DEHP was subsequently discontinued as a plasticizer after a great deal of concern was raised [13]. With the advancement of technology, we are able to detect trace amounts of chemicals in human tissue and analyze observations at the molecular level, thus systemic toxicity study will become more reliable.

Besides DEHP, silicone was also widely used in medical devices such as syringes, catheters, and implants. Unbelievably, Jean-Claude Mas of Poly Implant Prothese (PIP) used industrial-grade silicone in thousands of breast implants sold worldwide until December 2013, and some 300,000 women in 65 countries are believed to have received the faulty implants [15]. Industrial-grade silicone was not allowed be used to fabricate medical devices; however, for a higher profit margin, Poly Implant Prothese was willing to endanger people's health, exposing women to high rupture rate and high toxic risks. Prior to this event, three major suppliers of medical-grade silicone had already pulled out from the market in the 1990s due to fear of liability, because of litigations over silicone breast implants and unconfirmed immune-system disturbance. Under these conditions, a large number of important medical device products may become scarce resources and could even be unavailable on the market [13].

Other incidents involving biomaterials include toxic shock syndrome, latex allergies, and the use of talc on gloves, etc., which have emphasized the need for diligence in testing of biomaterials [16]. Biomaterials serve as basic raw materials for medical devices, which had a global market of $44 billion in 2012 [17]. Thus, the safeness of the biomaterial itself has a direct impact on the safety and effectiveness of resultant medical device products. Research on biomedical materials also helps to develop a wide range of applications of current biomaterials and even develop novel materials, such as nanobiomaterials which are gradually entering the market. The discussion on the safety of nanomaterials is always filled with controversies. In animal studies, carbon nanotubes were reported to be toxic to internal organs, but functionally modified carbon nanotubes were found to positively support cell adhesion and differentiation *in vitro*. The research and development of nanobiomaterials should consider investigating the full profile of their safety aspect in order to establish safe usage for medical devices with clinical relevance.

Besides raw materials, the design and manufacture processes are also crucial to the safety aspect of the product. Risk analysis, human factor, validation tests, and other related issues have to be taken into considerations. This will be further discussed in detail in Chapter 8.

Another point that should be taken into consideration should be cyber-security. This is especially so for those devices that require operating systems which include software or a mobile application. Operating systems are present in a vast number of medical devices, especially for major medical equipment. Usually, the operating systems are integral to the operation of the devices and would be considered a component of the device. A malfunction of an operating system can result in serious injury or even lead to death [18]. Remote access through the Internet was also observed to be on the rise as the Internet becomes more easily and readily accessible in our daily life, making it very convenient for patients and doctors to track the disease signals, but this also puts the patient's life at risk should a hacker override control.

1.4 The development of regulations and standards

Ideally, all stakeholders should cooperate to ensure the safety and effectiveness of medical devices by sharing responsibility, good communication, participation, education, and risk/cost assessment as illustrated in Figure 1.8 [19]. Governments should take the lead by establishing policies, regulations, and/or standards to create healthy cooperation among stakeholders. Table 1.5 and Figure 1.9 summarize the list of regulatory authorities and related device control and assessment in various countries which have comprehensive regulatory systems in place.

The most comprehensive regulatory system comes from the USFDA. The USFDA's budget was approximately $2 billion, approximately $45 million of which was allocated to the Center for Devices & Radiological Health (CDRH) activities in FY2009; the CDRH is in charge of medical devices [20]. The USFDA has had a

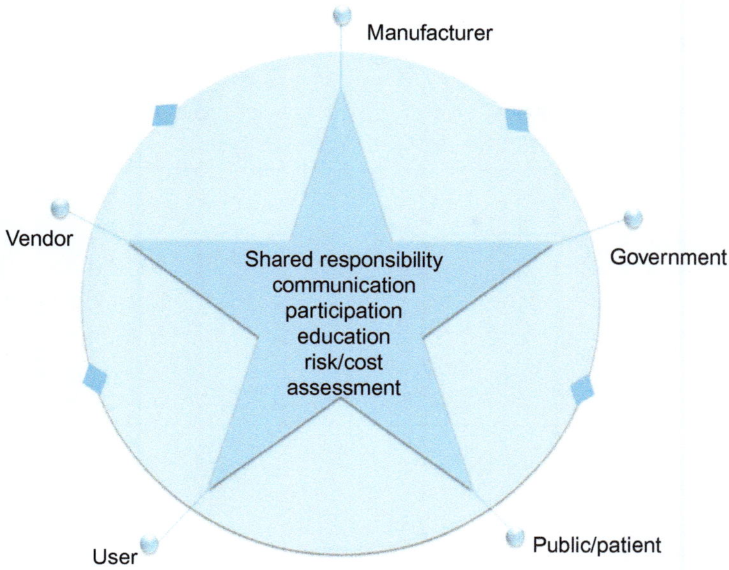

Figure 1.8 Ideal conditions for ensuring the safety and performance of medical devices by all stakeholders [19].

considerable increase in both responsibilities and resources to keep up with device development, as have other countries. Unfortunately, as of 2013, there are still 41% of 155 countries who still do not have national standards in place or recommended lists of medical devices for different types of healthcare facilities or specific procedures [21].

The regulations and standards should cover the whole life cycle of medical devices to ensure good practices (good laboratory practice, good clinical practice, and good manufacturing practice) as indicated in Figure 1.10. ISO has established and updated those standards corresponding to four related key aspects periodically, as illustrated in Figure 1.11. For example, ISO 13485 was derived from EN 46001, after that it was updated in 1996, 2003, and 2012. Standards only represent the requirements achievable by the current technological capabilities in the specific field, they should not hinder innovations and advancements. Thus, they must be reviewed regularly to remain in tune with technological advances.

Although most standards are voluntary, once the government includes them in their regulations, they become mandatory. Using the USFDA and the Singapore HSA as examples to compare with ISO standards, in Figure 1.12 we see the similarities and differences of those four aspects. As the manufacturer, strict adherence to regulatory requirements is essential but insufficient [13]. Compliance with the regulations and setting high standards and effective management systems will be crucial in ensuring the safety and effectiveness of the devices, protecting the patients and users, and preventing any adverse events from occurring.

Table 1.5 List of regulatory authorities and their controls on medical devices in various countries

Country	Regulatory authority	Product control	Key quality system regulations/standards	Conformity assessment
USA (United States of America)	Food & Drug Administration (FDA), Center for Devices & Radiological Health (CDRH)	PMA approval letter, Investigational Device Exemption (IDE) or 510(k) marketing clearance	21CFR820 cGMPs	Government
Canada	Therapeutic Products Directorate	Device licence	ISO 13485	Third Party
EU (European Union)	European Commission Directorate, Member state	Compliance label (CE mark)	Directive 90/385/EEC; Directive 93/42/EEC; Directive 98/79/EEC; ISO 13485	Third Party
Japan	Ministry of Health, Labour & Welfare (MHLW) through Pharmaceuticals & Medical Devices Agency (PMDA)	Approval or Notification to grant Manufacture licence, import licence, or sales notification respectively	Pharmaceutical Administration Law (PAL)	Government & Third Party
Australia	Therapeutic Goods Administration (TGA)	ARTG No.	ISO 13485?	Government & Third Party
China	China Food & Drug Administration (CFDA)	Medical Device Registration Certificate	ISO 13485 YY/T0287 GMP regulations	Government
India	Drug Controller General of India (DCGI) Central Drugs Standard Control Organization (CDSCO)	Registration Certificate (RC) Product Registration approval by the USFDA or in GHTF countries and the CE mark are recognized.	ISO 13485 Drugs & Cosmetics Act 1940 (Act) Drugs & Cosmetics Rules 1945	Government
Singapore	Health Science Authority (HSA)	Approval	GN-01~GN-31, ISO 13485	Government

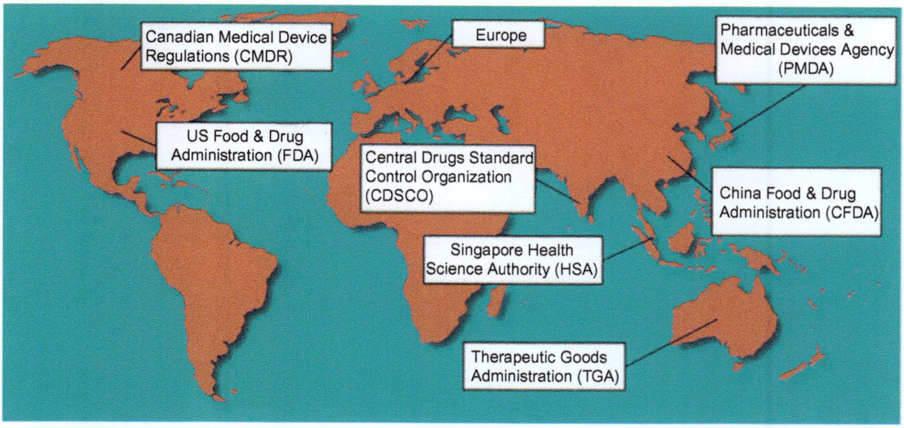

Figure 1.9 Regulatory authorities in various countries (United States, Canada, Europe, India, Singapore, Australia, China, and Japan).

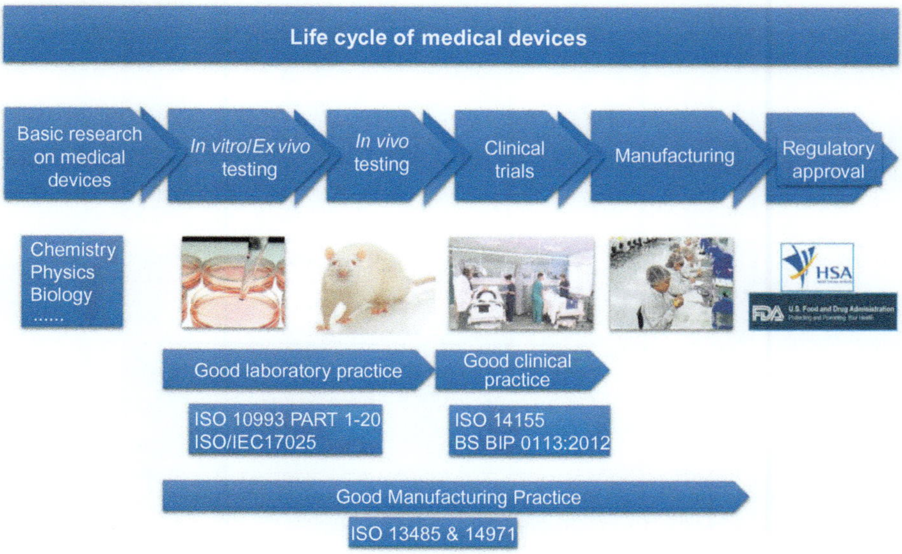

Figure 1.10 Life cycle of medical devices from research and development until regulatory approval.

1.5 The structure of this book

Figure 1.10 has schematically described the life cycle of medical devices. This book will address those key stages of the life cycle accordingly in three parts (Part I–III).

In Part I, we will be covering topics on the regulation of medical devices in various countries, management systems, standards for medical device manufacture, and the

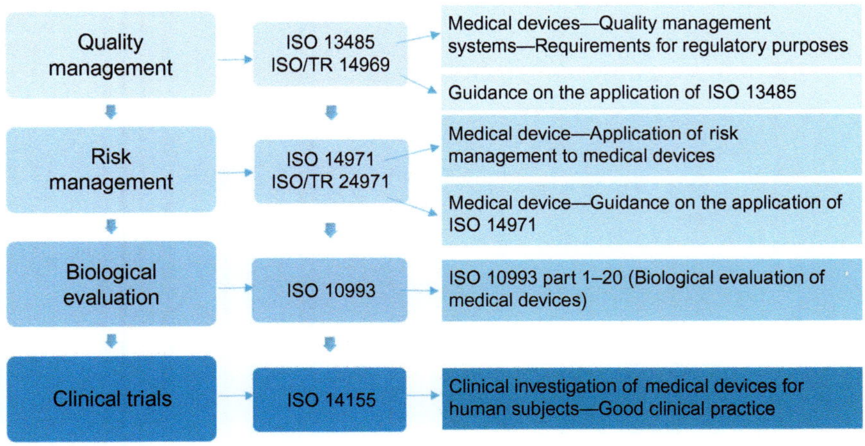

Figure 1.11 ISO Standards for medical devices.

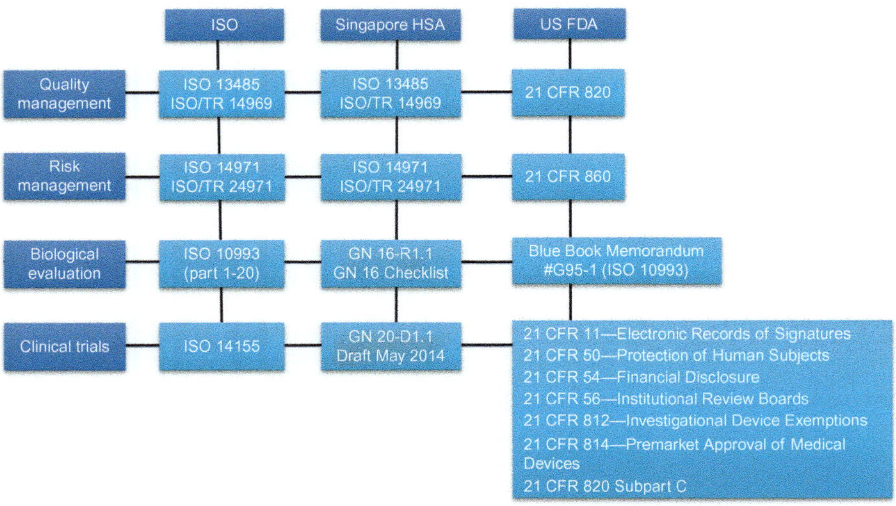

Figure 1.12 Standards and regulations on medical devices.

process of gaining approval for new medical devices. In addition, we have compiled recent changes to the regulations and standards.

In Part II, we will provide guidance on risk assessment procedures for a new medical device, safety testing and clinical testing of a new medical device based on three main ISO standards, namely ISO 14971, ISO 10993, and ISO 14155, as well as other critical standards or guidelines. Based on the latest version of those standards, we illustrate the current state of the standards and guidance documents.

In Part III, we will discuss the practices including product design overview and case studies and will highlight the role of the international medical device regulator forum in the global harmonization. Most medical devices are used globally, thus the harmonization of medical device regulations and standards is critical [19].

After each chapter, FAQs provide some brief questions and answers to quickly address beginners' doubts. At the end, references and important links are listed for further reading and future update.

The book is an excellent resource for biomedical engineering students and medical device professionals. We also wish to shed light on the importance of regulations and standards among all stakeholders, bioengineering designers, biomaterial scientists, or researchers co-developing a brighter future including medical devices for sustainable human life.

FAQs

(1) Which of the organizations and their standards should I adhere to for a medical device?
You should follow the standard which your country is using. If you intend to market your products in the EU or the United States, then you will need to follow EU and US FDA regulations, respectively.

(2) Is there a single entity that controls all the different regulatory authorities in the different countries?
There is an international medical device regulator forum; however it does not enforce a single standard for all countries.

(3) How are devices determined to belong to the higher risk group?
This is usually determined by the regulatory authority of the country.

(4) What are some of the devices that are provided in combination with drugs?
Devices that are provided in combination with drugs could be anything from your household simple medicated adhesive bandages commonly found in first aid boxes and pharmacy to complex pacemakers which require invasive surgery.

(5) What should I do if my device is not listed in the ISO?
The exact device may not be listed, it could be classified or grouped together with another device. The applicant would have to check with their regulatory authority for confirmation.

(6) How can a medical device improve the quality of life?
A medical device may return an ability to someone who has lost it. For example, prosthetics for the physically disabled or a pacemaker may return a partial or full ability that a patient previously lost.

(7) What are some of the adverse reporting systems available?
The FDA Adverse Event Reporting System (FAERS) for the United States, The Canada Vigilance Program, and the national spontaneous adverse event (AE) monitoring system administered by the Singapore Health Sciences Authority (HSA) are some of these systems.

(8) Who does the conformity assessment for Canada and the European Union?
Conformity Assessment Bodies of Canada are available on http://www.ic.gc.ca/eic/site/ceb-bhst.nsf/eng/h_tt00039.html. For Information regarding certification bodies send to cb.inquiries@ic.gc.ca. For European Union, see http://ec.europa.eu/enterprise/newapproach/nando/index.cfm?fuseaction=country.main for the list of notified bodies in the respective countries.

(9) If most standards are voluntary, why does a government include them in the regulations?
Most standards were set as a minimum requirement to ensure the safety of the products. These standards have to be met to safeguard the welfare of the users.

Part One

Regulations and standards

General regulations of medical devices

2

2.1 Introduction

The objectives of regulatory controls are to safeguard the health and safety of patients and users by ensuring that manufacturers of medical devices follow specified procedures during the design, manufacture, and marketing of the medical device. Globally, medical devices are classified into three or four categories by level of risk, and the regulatory controls are proportional to the level of risk associated with the medical device accordingly. To regulate the medical device market, there is a need to classify medical devices based on the potential risk to patients and users.

Figure 2.1 shows the general concept of how medical devices are classified by the level of risk. The same category in different countries may not be equivalent.

The risk level of a medical device is attributed by a series of factors, including: the duration of the device's contact with the body; the degree of the invasiveness; whether the device is implantable or active; and whether or not the device contains a substance, which in its own right is considered to be a medicinal substance and has action ancillary to that of the device. Table 2.1 indicates how the risk level of a medical device is determined principally. But in practice, the classification is a more complex process for each country.

Generally, there are national healthcare policies and/or laws and regulations set in place to regulate medical devices in each country, and harmonized standards also could be used as references. The hierarchy of regulatory requirements in various countries is shown in Table 2.2. In this chapter, we will review the regulations for medical devices in various countries, such as the United States, the EU, China, Japan, Australia, India, and Singapore. The regulatory authority, the classification of medical devices, and the controls will be introduced in this chapter.

2.2 The United States

2.2.1 The regulatory authority for medical devices and its organization in the United States

The Food and Drug Administration (FDA) is an agency within the United States (US) Department of Health and Human Services (HSS), which consists of the Office of the Commissioner, Office of Foods and Veterinary Medicine, Office of Global Regulatory Operations and Policy, Office of Medical Products and Tobacco, and Office of Operations. The Centre for Devices and Radiological Health (CDRH), which

Medical devices. http://dx.doi.org/10.1016/B978-0-08-100289-6.00002-8

Country/ organization	Classification			
US	Class I	Class II		Class III
EU	Class I	Class IIa	Class IIb	Class III
China	Class I	Class II		Class III
Japan	Class I	Class II	Class III	Class IV
Australia	Class I	Class IIa	Class IIb	Class III
Singapore	Class A	Class B	Class C	Class D
Risk	Low risk	Low-moderate risk	Moderate-high risk	High risk

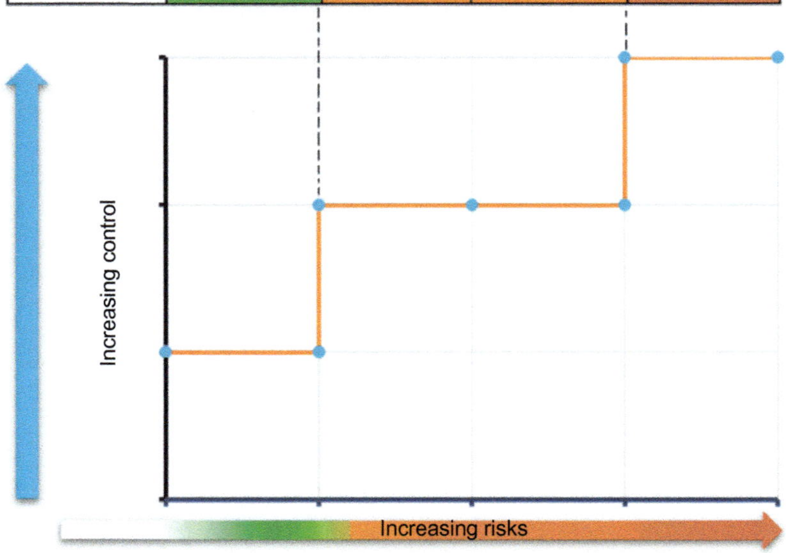

Figure 2.1 The classification of medical devices by level of risk and the regulatory controls in different countries.

Table 2.1 The basic principles for determining the risk of medical devices

	Transient	Short term	Long term
Noninvasive	Low	Low	Medium
Invasive	Low	Medium	High
Implantable	Medium	High	High

Table 2.2 Hierarchy of regulatory requirements in various countries

	General	United States	EU	China	Japan	Australia	India	Singapore
Level 1	Act	Food, Drug, and Cosmetic Act	Directive 90/385/ EEC; 93/42E EC; 98/79 EC	Drug Administration Law of the People's Republic of China	Act on Securing Quality, Efficacy and Safety of Pharmaceuticals, Medical Devices, Regenerative and Cellular Therapy Products, Gene, Therapy Products, and Cosmetics (previously referred as pharmaceutical affairs law)	Therapeutic Good Act 1989	The Drugs and Cosmetics Act 1940; The Drugs and Cosmetics (4th Amendment) Rules, 2010	Health Products Act (2007)
Level 2	Regulation	Regulations under CFR title 21, e.g., Quality System Regulations (21 CFR 820)		Regulation on the Supervision and Administration of Medical Devices (2014)		Therapeutic Good (Medical Devices) Regulations 2002		Health Products (Medical Devices) Regulations 2010

Continued

Table 2.2 Continued

	General	United States	EU	China	Japan	Australia	India	Singapore
Level 3	Guidance document/ standard	Recognized standards: http://www.accessdata.fda.gov/scripts/cdrh/cfdocs/cfStandards/search.cfm; Guidance documents: http://www.fda.gov/MedicalDevices/DeviceRegulationandGuidance/GuidanceDocuments/default.htm	Guidelines: http://ec.europa.eu/health/medical-devices/documents/guidelines/index_en.htm	Normative documents: http://www.sfda.gov.cn/WS01/CL1102/ (available in Chinese)	Certification standards, approval standards and review guideline: http://www.std.pmda.go.jp/stdDB/index_e.html	Australian regulatory guidelines for medical devices (ARGMD) and other guidelines: https://www.tga.gov.au/standards-guidelines-publications-medical-devices-ivds	Guidance documents: http://www.cdsco.nic.in/forms/contentpagel.aspx?lid=1674	Guidance documents: http://www.hsa.gov.sg/content/hsa/en/Health_Products_Regulation/Medical_Devices/Overview/Guidances_for_Medical_Device_Registration.html

regulates the design, manufacture, repackage, relabel, and/or import of medical devices into the United States, is found under the Office of Medical Products and Tobacco (Figure 2.2). Within the CDRH, at the top of the organization chart is the Office of Centre Director, which includes the CDRH Ombudsman, followed by seven offices. The United States has a centralized and comprehensive system to regulate medical devices, in which the FDA plays a central role as a regulator.

2.2.2 Classification of medical devices and the relevant controls in the United States

Before going into the legal aspects of registering a medical device, it is crucial to verify the product is indeed considered to be a medical device according to US CODE Title 21—Food and Drugs, Subchapter II—Definitions, Section 321, which is equivalent to the Federal Food, Drug, and Cosmetic Act (FD&C Act) Section 201, which defines "Medical Device" (Table 1.1 of Chapter 1). This definition also distinguishes medical devices from drugs, biological products, and other regulated products. To check whether your product is a medical device, you can search using the link provided below: http://www.accessdata.fda.gov/scripts/cdrh/cfdocs/cfpcd/classification.cfm.

The FDA classifies medical devices into three levels of risk posed to the patient and with which the device is associated; namely Class I to III, with Class I being the lowest in risk and Class III having the greatest risk (Figure 2.3). Class I medical devices are the lowest in risk and an example would be a cane or a walking stick. Class II medical devices are moderate in risk; higher than Class I but lower than Class III; an example of which is an acupuncture needle. Class III medical devices are the highest in risk and an example would be an automated external defibrillator.

There are various regulatory controls for medical devices in the United States, the descriptions and applications of the regulatory controls, such as General Controls [22, 23] and Special Controls [23], exemptions, such as Class I/II exemptions [24], 510(k) [25], and PMA [23, 26] are shown in Table 2.3 and Figure 2.4.

Regulatory controls are also in line with the three classes of medical devices. This means that the higher the class in which the device is grouped, the more regulatory control/paper work is required. Fundamentally, all medical devices are regulated by the General Controls regardless of their class, unless exempted. As seen in Figure 2.3, Class I devices are controlled by General Controls (such as tests of sterility) and may require Premarket Notification (PMN) [510(k)] before they are marketed; however, most of the devices are exempted from 510(k) because of lower risk concern. There are about 780 device types under Class I and only about 50 device types require the 510(k). Class II has additional controls; Special Controls apart from General Controls, and will usually require a 510(k). Class III has the highest level of regulatory control which requires Premarket Approval (PMA) before the device can be marketed.

General Controls provide the basis for regulating the three classes of medical devices, but they apply typically to Class I devices. Class I devices are not intended to be used for supporting or sustaining life or preventing impairment to human life and

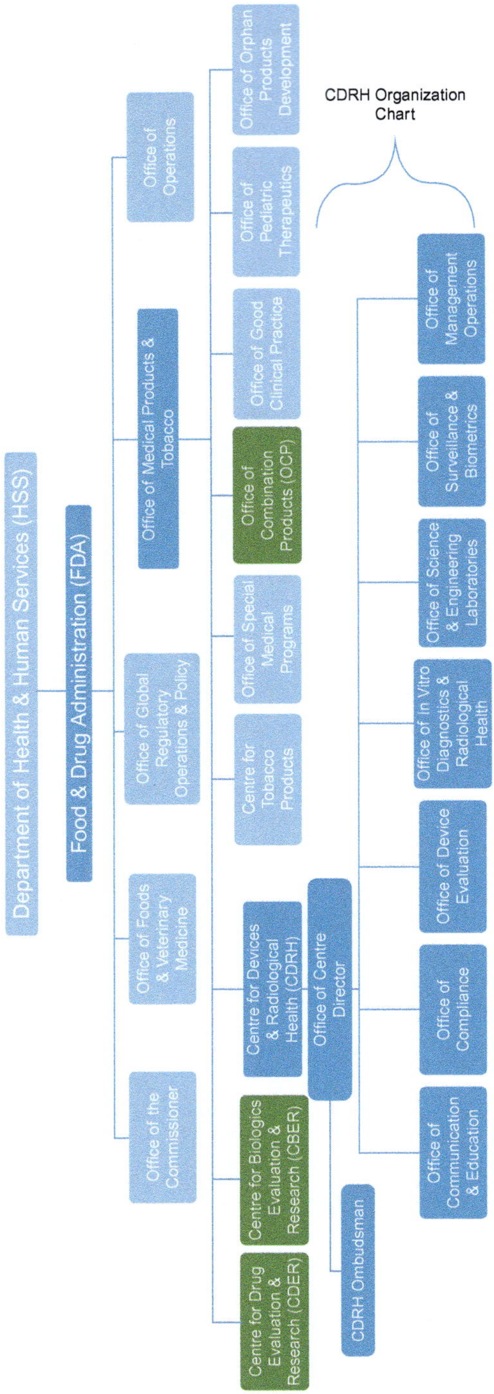

Figure 2.2 The organization of the USFDA.

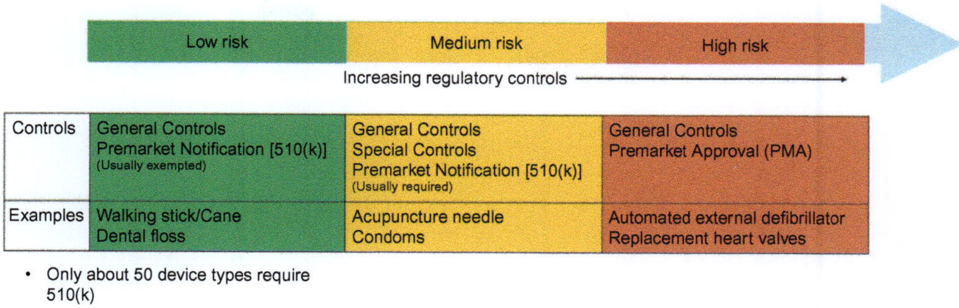

Figure 2.3 Classifying types of medical device by level of risk in the United States.

Table 2.3 The regulatory controls towards medical devices in the United States

Regulatory controls	Descriptions
General controls	General controls are regulatory requirements authorized by the FD&C Act, under section 501, 502, 510, 516, 518, 519, and 520, and they apply to all medical devices, unless exempted by regulations [22, 23].
Special controls	Special controls are regulatory requirements for Class II devices, for which general controls alone are insufficient to provide reasonable assurance of the safety and effectiveness of the device. Special controls are usually device-specific and include: performance standards, postmarket surveillance, patient registries, special labeling requirements, premarket data requirements, and guidelines [23].
Class I/II exemptions	Most Class I devices and a few Class II device are exempt from 510(k) requirements subject to the limitations on exemptions. However, these devices are not exempt from other general controls. A few Class I devices are additionally exempt from the GMP requirements with the exception of complaint files and general record keeping requirements [24].
Premarket notification (510(k))	Each person who wants to market in the United States, a Class I, II, III device intended for human use, for which a premarket approval (PMA) is not required, must submit a 510(k) to FDA unless the device is exempt from the 510(k) requirements. A 510(k) is a premarket submission to FDA to demonstrate that the device to be marketed is at least safe and effective, that is, substantially equivalent, to a legally marketed device that is not subject to PMA [25].
Premarket approval (PMA)	PMA is a FDA process of scientific and regulatory review to evaluate the safety and effectiveness of Class III medical devices. PMA is the most stringent type of device marketing application required by FDA. The applicant must receive FDA approval of its PMA application prior to marketing the device [23, 26].

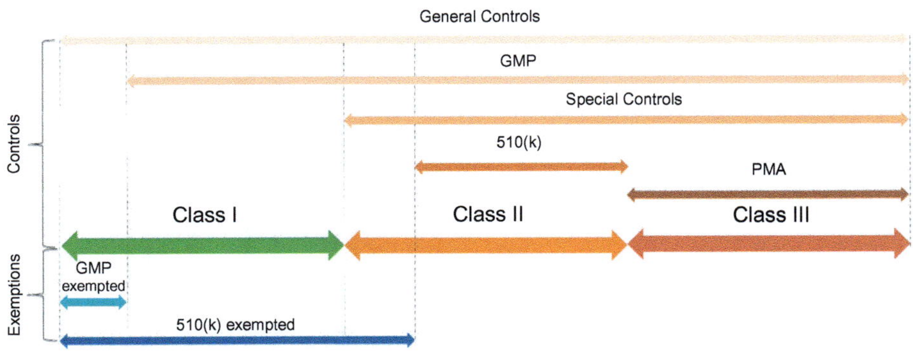

Figure 2.4 The regulatory controls and exemptions for medical devices in the United States.

may not present a potential unreasonable risk of illness or injury. Besides the General Controls, there are two other types of regulatory controls; 510(k) (also known as PMN), and PMA. Low risk Class I medical devices require the least regulatory controls; hence, they are mostly exempted from 510(k) or otherwise stated in the Code of Federal Regulations (CFR). Class II devices usually require 510(k), although some are exempted, and Class III requires PMA. The regulatory controls will be covered in more depth later.

One approach in the 510(k) submission demonstrates the device is "substantially equivalent" to a legally marketed device. Substantially equivalent means:

(1) the same intended use as the predicate device;
(2) the same technological characteristics as the predicate device; or
(3) has different technological characteristics but is as safe and effective as a legally marketed device; and
(4) does not raise different questions of safety and effectiveness than the predicate device.

To safeguard the public health after the device is on the market, the FDA requires a range of postmarket surveillance activities, including adverse event reporting and postmarket studies, to ascertain and monitor the device's safety and effectiveness.

2.2.3 Practical guide to identifying the medical devices classification in the United States

In the United States, every device is assigned a panel, and the panel determines the class and other controls and exemptions. The outcome is a regulation that specifies the classification, controls, and exemptions [27]. There are two methods for accomplishing this: go directly to the *Classification database* (http://www.accessdata.fda.gov/scripts/cdrh/cfdocs/cfpcd/classification.cfm) and search for a part of the device name, or, if you know the *device panel (medical specialty)* to which your device belongs, go directly to the listing for that panel (http://www.fda.gov/MedicalDevices/DeviceRegulationandGuidance/Overview/ClassifyYourDevice/ucm051530.htm) and identify your device and the corresponding regulation.

The FDA categorizes and organizes over 1700 distinct medical devices into Medical Speciality "Panels." These panels are documented in Title 21 of the Code of Federal Regulations (21 CFR), Parts 862–892. The 21 CFR 862–892 provides a detailed description of the device, how it is used, its classification, and other details regarding limitations of exemptions from section 510(k). For example, using two different methods for searching "Skull punch," the final information you can get is shown in Figure 2.5.

The example of a Class I medical device is a cane, or walking stick (Figure 2.6). It can be found classified under Physical Medicine panel, Part 890, Section 890.3075, and it is exempted from PMN [510(k)]. Any limitations of this exemption will be stated under 21 CFR xxx.9, where xxx refers to Parts 862–892; in this case, 21 CFR 890.9. The cane is one of a few Class I devices that have been exempted from Good Manufacturing Practice (GMP) requirements.

The acupuncture needle, which is a Class II medical device, requires Special Controls as listed in the 21 CFR below, as well as additional requirements listed in the section for *Prescription Devices* (21 CFR 801.109) (Figure 2.7). This has to be compliant in order to submit a PMN [510(k)]. PMA is usually not required for a Class II medical device.

The automated external defibrillator is a Class III medical device and it requires PMA (Figure 2.8). Additional requirements are listed in *Effective dates of requirement for premarket approval* (21 CFR 870.3).

In summary, some regulatory issues for medical devices in the United States are highlighted here:

(1) The medical devices are classified into Class I, Class II, and Class III, and the classification is determined by the USFDA;
(2) Controls are subject to the classification;
(3) For the devices which are substantially equivalent to the existing device, 510(k) is applied;
(4) For new devices, PMA is applied to demonstrate the device is safe and effective.

2.3 The European Union

2.3.1 Regulatory framework for medical devices in the EU

The EU was not always as big as it is today, and over time, more and more countries decided to join. The union reached its current size of 28 member countries with the accession of Croatia on July 1, 2013. The member countries and the year of entry are [28]:

> Austria (1995), Belgium (1952), Bulgaria (2007), Croatia (2013), Cyprus (2004), Czech Republic (2004), Denmark (1973), Estonia (2004), Finland (1995), France (1952), Germany (1952), Greece (1981), Hungary (2004), Ireland (1973), Italy (1952), Latvia (2004), Lithuania (2004), Luxembourg (1952), Malta (2004), Netherlands (1952), Poland (2004), Portugal (1986), Romania (2007), Slovakia (2004), Slovenia (2004), Spain (1986), Sweden (1995), and United Kingdom (1973).

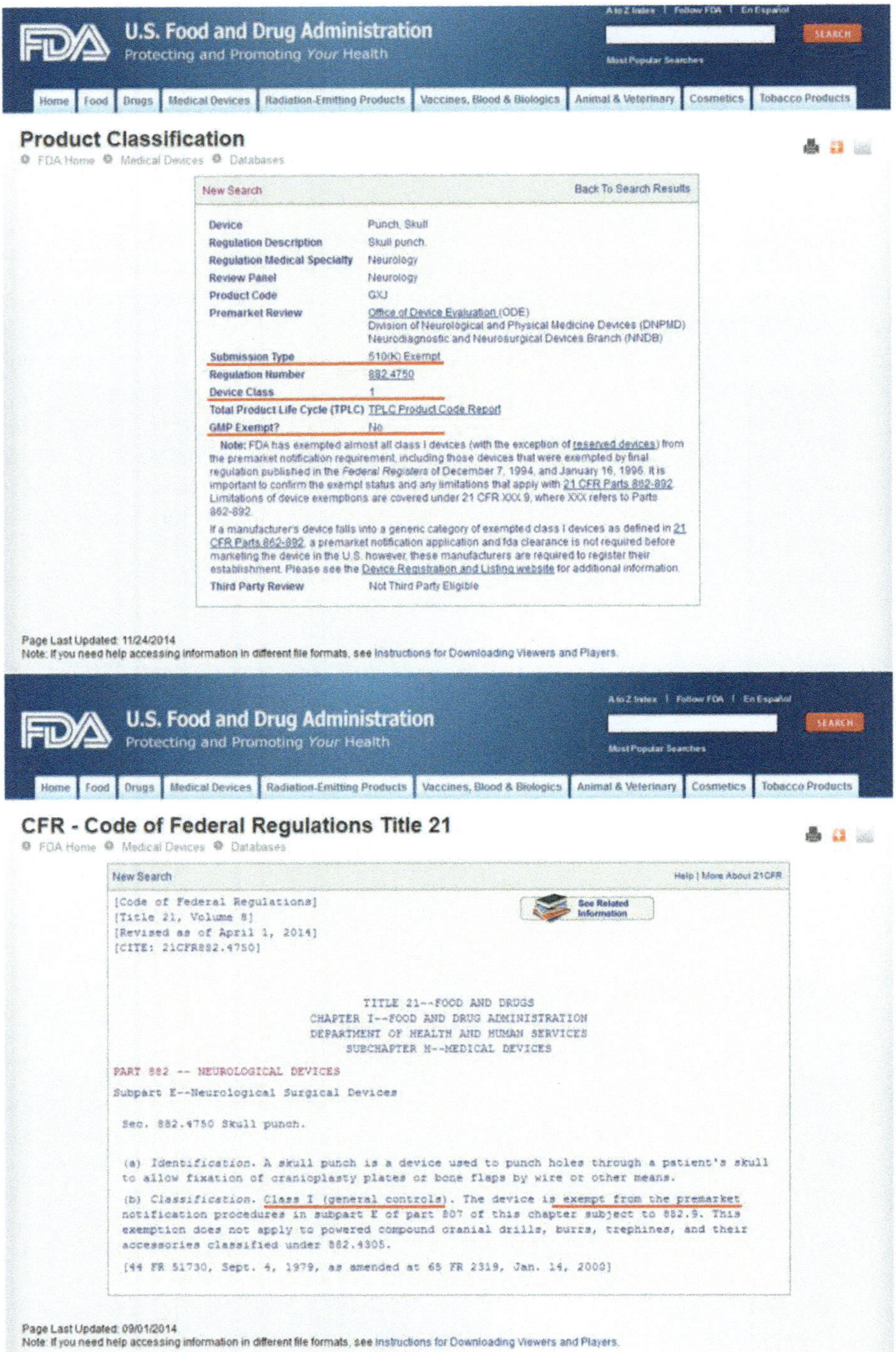

Figure 2.5 Using classification database and medical specialty for searching for a medical device.

Class I

[CITE 21CFR890.3075]

Sec.890.3075Cane.

(a) *Identification. A cane is a device intended for medical purposes that is used to provide minimal weight support while walking. Examples of canes include the following: A standard cane, a forearm cane, and a cane with a tripod, quad or retractable stud on the ground end.*

(b) *Classification. Class I (general controls). The device is exempt from the premarket notification procedures in subpart E of part 807 of this chapter, subject to the limitations in 890.9. The device is also exempt from the current good manufacturing practice requirements of the quality system regulation in part 820 of this chapter, with the exception of 820.180, regarding general requirements concerning records and 820.198, regarding complaint files.*

[48 FR 53047, Nov. 23, 1983, as amended at 66 FR 38816, July 25, 2001]

Figure 2.6 21CFR890.3075.

ClassII

[CITE21CFR880.5580]

Sec.880.5580Acupunctureneedle

(a) *Identification. An acupuncture needle is a device intended to pierce the skin in the practice of acupuncture. The device consists of a solid, stainless steel needle. The device may have a handle attached to the needle to facilitate the delivery of acupuncture treatment.*

(b) *Classification. Class II (special controls). Acupuncture needles must comply with the following special controls:*

(1) *Labeling for single use only and conformance to the requirements for prescription devices set out in 21 CFR 801.109.*

(2) *Device material biocompatibility, and*

(3) *Device sterility*

[61 FR 64617, Dec. 6, 1996]

Figure 2.7 21CFR880.5580.

Class III

[CITE 21CFR870.5310]

Sec. 870.5310 Automatedexternal defibrillator

(a) *Identification. An automated external defibrillator (AED) is a low-energy device with a rhythm recognition detection system that delivers into a 50 ohm test load an electrical shock of a maximum of 360 joules of energy used for defibrillating (restoring normal heart rhythm) the atria or ventricles of the heart. An AED analyses the patient's electrocardiogram, interprets the cardiac rhythm, and automatically delivers an electrical shock (fully automated AED), or advises the user to deliver the shock (semi-automated or shock advisory AED) to treat ventricular fibrillation pulseless ventricular tachycardia.*

(b) *Classification. Class III (premarket approval)*

(c) *Date PMA or notice of PDP is required. No effective date has been established of the requirement for premarket approval. See 870.3.*

[68 FR 61344, Oct. 28, 2003; 69 FR 10615, Mar. 8, 2004]

Figure 2.8 21CFR870.5310.

The EU does not have a government organization equivalent to the USFDA. In Europe, the regulatory bodies for medical devices are European Commission, National Competent Authority, and Notified Bodies (NBs). Manufacturers may interact with the latter two only when they plan to place medical devices on the European market, while European Commission does not directly interact with manufacturers, but rather acts as an overall coordinating body [29]. Until the 1990s, each member state had its own approach to regulate devices. To regulate the diverse and complex market and improve the internal market in Europe, medical device directives were introduced by the European Council that defined the essential requirements (ER) to ensure a devices' safety and performance [30]. Based on the new approach, rules relating to the safety and performance of medical devices were harmonized in the EU in the 1990s. The core legal framework consists of three directives:

(1) Directive 90/385/EEC (regarding active implantable medical devices);
(2) Directive 93/42/EEC (regarding medical devices);
(3) Directive 98/79/EC (regarding *in vitro* diagnostic medical devices).

These three main directives have been supplemented over time by several modifying and implementing directives, including the last technical revision brought by Directive 2007/47/EC.

Similar to those in the United States, the regulator controls over medical devices increase with the degree of risk associated with the device. Manufacture of low-risk (Class I) devices is required only to self-declare conformity with the ER to a National Competent Authority, such as the Medicines and Healthcare Products Regulatory Agency (MHRA) in the United Kingdom and the French Agency for the Safety of Health Products. Other devices (Class IIa, IIb, and III) require a combination of clinical and nonclinical data on the device being evaluated. If available, data for an equivalent device already on the market may be submitted. Manufacturers of these devices select NB to evaluate their devices and receive a CE mark. The CE marking symbolizes the conformity of the product with the applicable European Community requirements imposed on the manufacturer. The CE markings are affixed to products that conform to all applicable European Community provisions and indicate that the appropriate conformity assessment procedures have been completed. The declaration of conformity is the final step in the relevant conformity assessment procedure for all medical devices which fall under the scope of one of each of the directives and is incumbent to the manufacturer: in this step, the manufacturer ensures and declares that the products concerned meet the provisions of the directives. The declaration of conformity is a mandatory document which must imperatively be established and signed before any product release for sale and which must be kept at the regulators disposal. Once the device is on the market, the manufacturer is required to report all serious adverse events to the Competent Authority (CA). In Europe, this information is collated into a central database, the European Databank on Medical Devices (Eudamed). Eudamed contains data on manufacturers, certificate issues, modifications, suspensions, withdrawals, refusals, and clinical investigations. The use of Eudamed has been mandatory since 2011 [31]. The process is shown in Figure 2.9.

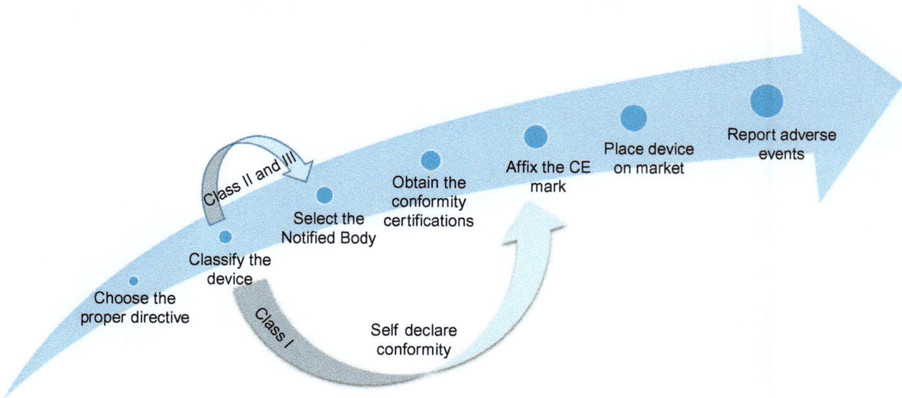

Figure 2.9 The route to comply with the regulatory requirements for a medical device manufacturer in the EU.

2.3.2 New changes in EU regulation

Since 2008, revision of the medical device directives has been initiated. Considering the premarket review, postmarket monitoring and surveillance, and information provision on devices and regulatory process, the weakness in European medical device regulations does exist, for example, no uniform standards and evidence requirements across Notified Body (premarket review). To address this issue, greater harmonization of the process and evidence standards will be utilized by Notified Body [31].

On 26 September 2012, the European Commission adopted a proposal for the regulation of the European parliament and of the council on medical devices and a proposal for a regulation of the European parliament and of the Council on *in vitro* diagnostic medical devices which will, once adopted by the European Parliament and by the Council, replace the existing three medical devices directives [32]. And the proposal was amended by the Parliament in October 2013 [33]. The motivation for the new proposals may come from the scandals, such as the one in which the French supplier Poly Implant Prostheses (PIP) had used a low-grade agricultural silicone in its artificial breast and got harmful medical devices approved by regulators in some of the east European member states [34].

All of the current legislation regulating medical devices is in the process of revision at the European level. This will replace the existing three European directives with two European regulations as Figure 2.10 indicates.

The new directives/regulations for medical devices have yet to be issued, and the expected changes are shown in Figure 2.11. The upcoming changes can be summarized in two aspects [35,36]:

(1) Extended
- Extension of the scope of EU legislation on medical devices to include implants for esthetic purposes, and clarified as regards genetic tests;

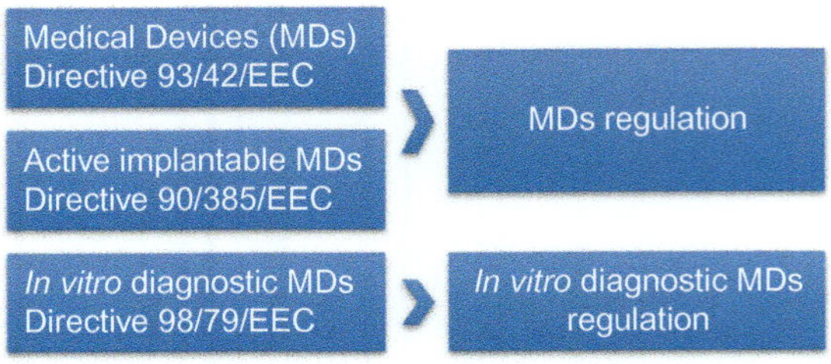

Figure 2.10 The changes of existing directives to regulations for medical devices in the EU.

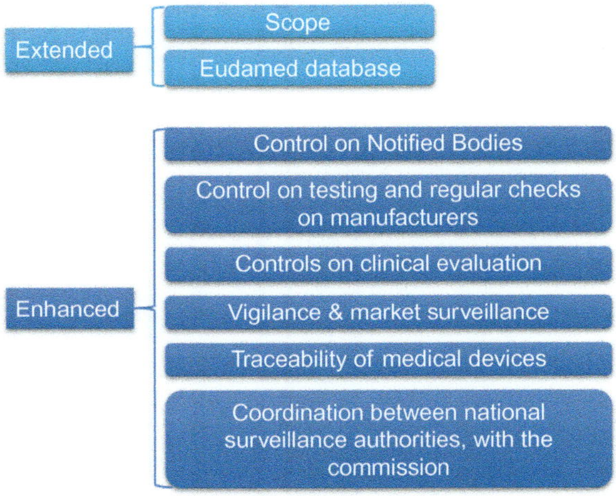

Figure 2.11 The expected changes in the upcoming medical device regulations in Europe.

- Eudamed database on medical devices will be extended to provide more comprehensive information on products available on the EU market. Nonconfidential data will be made available to public.

(2) Enhanced
- NB will continue to grant market approval through CE certification but will face increased oversight and assurance by the Competent Authorities and a new Medical Device Coordination Group (MDCG), especially for high-risk devices;
- Thorough testing and regular checks on manufacturers will be ensured through unannounced factory inspections—random, absolutely no prior notice and not conducted like scheduled QMS audit;
- Stricter requirements for clinical evidence to support assessments of medical devices;
- Duties and functions of manufacturer as well as member states will be redefined for the vigilance activities; the rights and the obligations of national Competent Authorities will be clarified to reinforce market surveillance;
- Better traceability of medical devices throughout the supply chain, enabling a swift and effective response to safety problems (e.g., recalls);
- Better coordination between national surveillance authorities and the Commission which is providing scientific, technical, and logistic support.

The new regulations on medical devices in Europe are yet to be released. We can, however, expect a better regulated medical device market in Europe after the adoption of the regulation. We believe that difficulties or controversies linked to the regulation implementation will also probably emerge in the next few years following the adoption.

In summary, the regulatory issues for medical devices in the EU are:

(1) The medical devices are classified into Class I, Class IIa, Class IIb, and Class III, and the classifications are determined by the manufacturer following a rule-based approach in Annex IX;
(2) Controls depend on the classification;
(3) No distinction between "existing" devices and "new" devices.

2.3.3 Differences between the regulations for medical devices in the United States and the EU

In the United States, the FDA oversees all regulations of medical devices. In contrast, the European system confers significant authority on a collection of governmental (Competent Authority [CA]) and private (Notified Body [NB]) bodies to oversee device evaluation, market approval, and postmarket surveillance. Table 2.4 summarizes the main differences between the United States and the EU for approval of medical devices [30].

2.4 China

2.4.1 The regulatory framework for medical devices in China

After more than three decades of effort, China has established a medical regulatory system from a nearly zero base, along with its national policy of reform and opening up of her market [37]. In China, China Food & Drug Administration (CFDA) is the regulatory authority for food, drugs, and medical devices. Under CFDA, the department of Medical Device Supervision takes on the responsibility for regulating medical devices. There are four divisions: general affairs, manufacturing supervision, distribution supervision, and monitoring and reevaluation. There are three levels of legislations in China, which are shown in Table 2.5.

The new regulations for the supervision and administration of medical devices (National Council Order No. 650) came into force as of October 1, 2014. The purpose of these regulations is to strengthen the supervision and administration of medical devices; to ensure their safety and effectiveness; and to protect human health, life, and safety. The regulations also include explanations of the administration of production, distribution, and use of medical devices as well as supervision and penalties in case of violation of the regulations [38]. The classification of medical devices and the relevant regulatory authorities in China [39] are shown in Table 2.6.

China has its own national standards (in the Chinese language), which follows the international standards closely, to regulate the medical devices market, as shown in the Table 2.7.

Table 2.4 Main differences for approval of medical devices between United States and European Union [30]

System feature	United States	European Union	Potential implications
Mandate	Oversight of public health	Device safety (overseen through Competent Authorities), device approval (through Notified Bodies), and facilitation of trade	May influence dealings with industry clients, and attention paid to balance between effectiveness and risk of safety concerns
Centralization	Oversight of all device regulation by the FDA	Directives outline processes carried out by Competent Authorities and Notified Bodies	Standardization and coordination of premarketing and postmarketing evaluation are theoretically simpler and easier to enforce in the United States
Data requirements	Reasonable assurance of safety and effectiveness for approval of high-risk devices, “substantially equivalence” for 510(k) clearance	Generally performance-based analysis, requiring proof that device works as intended	EU assessment made by manufacturers and Notified Bodies; provides less insight into clinical end points for high-risk devices
Transparency	Proprietary limits with public reporting of premarketing review of approved devices, recalls, and adverse events	Review of Notified Bodies not made public; postmarketing data shared among Competent Authorities but not with the public	Greater public access to evidence in the United States
Funding	Combination of federal appropriations (80%) and user fees (<20%)	Funding of Competent Authorities variable among countries; Notified Bodies paid directly by sponsors	Notified Bodies may be vulnerable to conflict of interest with industry client; the FDA may be influenced by changes in federal funding and political climate
Access	Clinical premarketing testing of high-risk devices delays patient access to these devices (no differences for low- and moderate-risk devices)	EU patients may have access to certain high-risk devices sooner than in the United States, subject to limitations by payers	EU patients have faster access to certain devices, but these products are marketed with less rigorous proof of effectiveness and may have a greater chance of later-identified adverse events

Table 2.5 Legislation on medical devices in China

Three levels of legislation	Function
Regulations for the supervision and administration of medical deceives	National regulations
CFDA orders	Provide the detail for implementing the regulations
Normative documents of the central or local FDAs	Similar to standards

Table 2.6 Classification, definition, and the regulatory authority of medical devices in China [39]

Classification	Definition	Regulatory authority
Class I	Safety and effectiveness can by ensured through routine administration	Domestic: Local FDA Import: CFDA
Class II	Further control administration is required to ensure safety and effectiveness	Domestic: Provincial FDA Import: CFDA
Class III	Implanted into human body, or used for life support of sustenance, or pose potential risk to human body and thus, must be strictly controlled in respect to safety and effectiveness	CFDA

Table 2.7 Medical devices related international standards and their equivalents in China

International standards	Equivalent in China
ISO 13485	YY/T0287
ISO 14971	YY/T0316
IEC 60601-1	GB 9706.1

2.4.2 Changes in Chinese regulations

2.4.2.1 The evolution of CFDA

Readers may have heard of "SFDA" before and may have wondered about its relationship with the CFDA. In recent years, the regulatory system and regulations in China has been reformed, and we will briefly introduce the changes in the following paragraph.

In China, medical devices regulation began in 1994 under the State Pharmaceutical Administration of China (SPAC). In 1998, the SPAC merged with the Department of Drugs Administration of the Ministry of Health (MOH) and formed the State Drug Administration (SDA). In 2003, many of the original functions of the Chinese

MOH were diverted to other departments and the SDA was renamed the State Food and Drug Administration (SFDA). In March of 2013, SFDA was restructured from the previous SFDA to the CFDA, which was announced in the decision made by State Council. Unless otherwise stated, all the documents and decisions released by the SFDA retain the validity for the CFDA.

In 2010, the Chinese government declared the Good Manufacturing Practice of Medical Devices (Interim GMP Regulations) and Good Manufacturing Practice of Medical Device Inspection (GMP Inspection Regulations), which went into effect in March of 2011. These regulate the methods, facilities, and controls for the "design, manufacture, packaging, labeling, storage, installation, and servicing of all finished devices intended for human use" [40].

2.4.2.2 Revised regulation on the supervision and administration of medical devices

In March 2014, the State Council of the Chinese Central Government unveiled a revised Regulation on the Supervision and Administration of Medical Devices (revised regulation, National Council Order No. 650). The revised regulation came into effect on June 1, 2014 and replaces the previous Regulation on the Supervision and Administration of Medical Devices issued by the Chinese government April 1, 2000 (original regulation, National Council Order No. 276). As a result of the rapid growth of the Chinese medical devices industry, the original regulation is no longer effective in addressing issues in the industry [41]. The revised regulation is more detailed, with a total of eight chapters, while the old one only had six chapters. The two newly added chapters focus on adverse event monitoring and product recall and supervision and inspections. Besides the added chapters, some changes [42, 43] to other chapters also can be tracked from different perspectives (Table 2.8).

Only the Chinese version of the New Regulations (National Council Order No. 650) is available through the CFDA official Website currently. The English version available on the Website is still the translation of the original Regulation (National Council Order No. 276), the old regulation. Because the new regulations just came into effect on June 1, 2014, and most of the relevant guidance documents, such as the CFDA orders, only came into effect on October 1, 2014, to the best of our knowledge, there are no examples for reference of who has gone through the process required by the new regulation and orders. We believe that there will be a transition period (one or two years, or even more) ahead. The changes made in the revised regulation demonstrate the Chinese Central Government's new efforts to improve and uphold a comprehensive and effective regulatory framework for the medical device industry in China. On the same day the revised regulation was released, CFDA sought public comments on a number of related draft rules covering medical device registration and filing, manufacturing, and distribution. Moreover, the CFDA has also published various draft rules governing products classification, inspection criteria for GMP, GSP (good supply practice) for distributors, and amendments for a number of product categories over the past months. It is anticipated that the official promulgation of these rules will facilitate the enforcement of the revised regulation.

Table 2.8 Comparison between original (No. 276) and new regulations (No. 650) on supervision and administration of medical devices

	No. 276 with effect from April 1, 2000	No. 650 with effect from June 1, 2014
Chapter I	Article 1-6: General Provisions	Article 1-7: General Provisions
Chapter II	Article 7-18: The administration of Medical Devices	Article 8-19: Registration & Filing for Medical Devices
Chapter III	Article 19-28: Administration of Production, Distribution, and Use of Medical Devices	Article 20-28: Production of Medical Devices
Chapter IV	Article 29-34: Supervision of Medical Devices	Article 29-45: Distribution & Use of Medical Devices
Chapter V	Article 35-46: Penalties	Article 46-52: Adverse Event Monitoring & Product Recall
Chapter VI	Article 47-48: Supplementary Provisions	Article 53-62: Supervision & Inspection
Chapter VII	NA	Article 63-75: Legal Liability
Chapter VIII	NA	Article 76-80: Supplementary Provisions

The changes mainly include the following four aspects:

(1) Optimized registration and approval process

For marketing medical devices, the review and approval process has been optimized including requirements such as Class I medical devices are only required for filing instead of registration, which is great news for manufacturers and distributors of medical devices.

(2) Stricter supervision on the production process

According to the new regulation, product registration certificates are required to be submitted for the application of a production permit for Class II and Class III medical devices. Previously, production permits were only required from a company before application for a product registration certificate.

(3) Simplified process on distribution and use

Filing is no longer required for the companies which are distributing Class I medical devices, and only distributors of Class II medical devices are required to file with the CFDA at the municipal level (article 30).

(4) Consolidated postmarketing supervision

Chapter V "Adverse Event Monitoring & Product Recall" is a newly added chapter, through which we can see that the CFDA aims to centralize all postmarketing supervision. Problematic medical devices in the market can be effectively identified and removed from the shelves; the manufacturing, sales, distribution, and use of unsafe medical devices in the market can be stopped.

The details of the changes [44,45] can be found in Table 2.9.

Table 2.9 The detailed changes between original and new regulations [44, 45]

Item	Original regulation	New regulation	Possible results
Filing	NA	Class I device	Shorter approval timeframes
COO approval	NA	Imported MDs	Stricter controls on imported MDs
Certificate renewal	Every 4 years	Every 5 years	Longer validity period
On-site audit	Not required	May be required for foreign manufacturers	More emphasis on quality management system compliance
CFDA fees	Not required	May be required	More expenses for obtaining CFDA approval
Legal agent and after sales agent	Both required	Only legal agent required	Legal agent has more responsibility
IVD registration	Testing and clinical trials can proceed in parallel	Testing must occur before clinical trials	Longer timeframe for IVD registration

COO: country of original.

Medical device companies doing business in China should keep a close watch on the development of the draft rules and the actual enforcement of the revised regulation because the changes will have significant implications on their operations in China. According to the new regulations, even the duration required for approval seems much shorter, 62.89% of 2248 professionals worldwide think that application or registration in China has become more difficult due to the new regulations released in 2014 and there is general uncertainty over which products require clinical trials in China [46]. From a regulatory compliance perspective, for year (2015) China was ranked highest in terms of which markets are most difficult for device manufacturers [46].

2.5 Japan

The pharmaceuticals and medical devices agency (PMDA) is the regulatory agency of Japan. It works together with the Ministry of Health, Labor and Welfare (MHLW). The PMDA conducts scientific reviews of marketing authorization applications of pharmaceuticals and medical devices, monitoring their postmarketing safety. The PMDA is also responsible for providing relief compensation to victims of adverse drug reactions and infections by pharmaceuticals or biological products.

In Japan, the medical devices are divided into Class I, Class II, Class III, and Class IV. Class I medical devices are defined as general medical devices extremely low risk to the human body, such as X-ray film. Approval of Class I medical devices is not required, but marketing notification is necessary. Class II medical devices are controlled medical devices designated by the Minister of Health, Labor, and Welfare, for which applicable certification standards are specified by the Minister low risk to the human body (certification by a registered certification body is required) or other controlled medical devices low risk to the human body. Class III medical devices are specially controlled medical devices medium risk to the human body, such as artificial bones. Class IV medical devices are specially controlled medical devices highly invasive to patients high risk to the human body, such as heart valves. For Class III and Class IV medical devices, the Minister's approval for the product is required [47].

To learn more about the Japanese approval system for medical devices, please refer to: http://www.pmda.go.jp/english/service/outline_s.html. They offer live-chat consultation services, such as clinical trial consultation, as well as providing advice on application materials. The contact information is shown as follows:

Office of International Programs
Pharmaceuticals and Medical Devices Agency
Shin-Kasumigaseki Building
3-3-2 Kasumigaseki, Chiyoda-ku
Tokyo 100-0013, Japan
Telephone: +81-(0)3-3506-9456
Facsimile: +81-(0)3-3506-9572
English site: http://www.pmda.go.jp/english/index.html

2.6 Australia

In Australia, medical devices are regulated by the Therapeutic Goods Administration (TGA). The Australian medical device regulatory requirements, which were implemented in 2002, were largely based on the European Council Medical Device Directive (MDD) 93/42/EEC. Since July 2010, *in vitro* diagnostic devices (IVDs) have also been regulated as a subset of medical devices.

As part of the Department of Health, the TGA safeguards and enhances the health of the Australian community through effective and timely regulation of therapeutic goods. The TGA is responsible for regulating the supply, import, export, manufacturing, and advertising of therapeutic goods [48].

The TGA regulates medical devices via the following platforms:

(1) Premarket assessment;
(2) Postmarket monitoring and enforcement of standards;
(3) Licensing of Australian manufacturers and verifying overseas manufacturers' compliance with the same standards as their Australian counterparts.

The classification of medical devices in Australia [49] is shown in Table 2.10.

Table 2.10 **The TGA medical device classification system [49]**

Medical device classifications	Examples
Class I	Elastic bandages, tongue depressors, cervical collars, slings, nonsterile dressings
Class IIa	X-ray films, intravenous tubing, contact lenses, catheters
Class IIb	Blood bags, dressings for severe wounds, condoms
Class III	Coronary artery probes, intrauterine contraceptive devices, medical devices that contain medicines, such as dressings with an antimicrobial agent
Active implantable medical devices	Pace makers, cochlear implants

From the Behind the News: the regulation of medical devices, 2011, Therapeutic Goods Administration, used by permission of the Australian Government, http://www.tga.gov.au/behind-news/regulation-medical-devices.

2.7 India

Central drugs standard control organization (CDSCO) has been organized to safeguard and enhance the public health by assuring the safety, efficacy, and quality of drugs, cosmetics, and medical devices in India. Currently, there are no separate medical device regulations in India, and there is a serious mixing of drug and device regulations. The medical regulations are evolving and the direction is that the medical device regulations would shape up in line with the Global Harmonization Task Force (GHTF) guidelines [50]. The Drugs and Cosmetics Act 1940 & Rules 1945 are currently applicable to drugs as well as medical devices. India recognizes ISO standards. Product registration approvals by the USFDA or in GHTF countries and the CE mark are also recognized.

To better regulate medical devices as a separate category from pharmaceutical products, the Drugs and Cosmetics (Amendment) Bill, 2013 will be redrafted in line with recommendations from the experts' panel [51].

2.8 Singapore

2.8.1 Regulatory framework for medical devices in Singapore

Singapore Health Science Authority (HSA), Medical Device Branch, is entrusted with regulating medical devices in Singapore. The HSA has adopted the new regulatory system based on the principles endorsed by the Global Harmonization Task Force (GHTF) with modification to suit the Singapore context. The HSA has also studied the medical device regulatory system in developed country counterparts, including the USFDA, the European Union, Canada's Medical Devices Bureau (MDB), Japan's Ministry of

Health, Labor and Welfare (MHLW), and Australia's Therapeutic Goods Administration (TGA) [52], which are also referred as Reference Agencies.

In 2002, HSA introduced the Voluntary Product Registration Scheme and postmarket monitoring and surveillance program for medical devices in the Singapore market. With the passage of the Health Products Act 2007 in February 2007, HSA implemented the Health Products (Medical Devices) Regulations to further tighten the control of medical devices in the local market.

The Health Products Regulation Group (HPRG) of HSA is the national regulatory authority for health products. HPRG ensures that drugs, innovative therapeutics, medical devices, and health-related products in Singapore are controlled and meet appropriate standards of safety, quality, and efficacy.

All product registration applications are to be submitted via the online Medical Device Information and Communication System (MEDICS). Upon successful submission, the application will be screened before it can be accepted for evaluation to ensure that there are no major deficiencies that would hinder the evaluation.

Medical devices may be classified into four risk classes (Table 1.2 of Chapter 1). Regulatory control for medical devices in Singapore was implemented in three phases [52], and the details are shown in Table 2.11.

Table 2.11 Implementation of regulatory controls for medical devices in Singapore

	Duration	Description
Phase 1	01.11.2007– 31.10.2008	Report adverse events to HSA within stipulated time frame; Notify HSA prior to the initiation of a product recall; Keep records of complaints and product distribution
Phase 2	01.11.2008– 09.08.2010	Start accepting applications for licensing of dealers of medical devices and registration of medical device products
Phase 3	Stage 1 10.08.2010– 31.12.2011	Unlicensed manufacturing, importation and wholesaling of medical device is prohibited; Class C and D medical devices (but excluding those medical devices currently licensed under the Radiation Protection Act by the Centre for Radiation Protection and Nuclear Science (CRPNS) of the National Environment Agency (NEA)) that are imported and supplied must meet one of the criteria below: Listed on the Singapore Medical Device Register (SMDR); Listed on the Transition List; or Authorized via one of the Authorization Routes
	Stage 2 01.01.2012–	Unless exempted from product registration, all medical devices, including class A and B medical devices, that are imported and supplied must meet one of the criteria below: Listed on the Singapore Medical Device Register (SMDR); Listed on the Transition List; or Authorized via one of the Authorization Routes

The content is accurate as of July 2015, please refer to HSA website for updated information.

2.8.2 Grouping of medical devices for production registration in Singapore

In Singapore, medical devices that can be grouped into one of the following six categories can be submitted in one product registration application and listing in the Singapore Medical Device Register (SMDR): SINGLE, FAMILY, IVD TEST KIT, SYSTEM, IVD CLUSTER, and GROUP [53]. The identification of each of these categories is shown in Table 2.12.

Table 2.12 The grouping of medical devices for production registration in Singapore

Category	Description	Examples
SINGLE	A medical device from a product owner identified by a medical device proprietary name with a specific intended purpose. It is sold as a distinct packaged entity and does not meet the criteria for a FAMILY, IVD TEST KIT, SYSTEM, IVD CLUSTER, or a GROUP.	Condoms that are sold in packages of 3, 12, and 144 can be registered as a SINGLE medical device.
FAMILY	A collection of medical devices and each medical device FAMILY member: is from the same product owner; is of the same risk classification class; has the same medical device proprietary name; has a common intended purpose; has the same design and manufacturing process; and has variations that are within the scope of the permissible variants.	Condoms that differ in color, size, and texture but are manufactured from the same material and manufacturing process and share a common intended purpose can be registered as a FAMIILY.
IVD TEST KIT	An IVD device that consists of reagents or articles that are: from the same product owner; intended to be used in combination to complete a specific intended purpose; sold under a single TEST KIT name or the labeling, instructions for use (IFU), brochures or catalogues for each reagents or article states that the component is intended for use with the IVD TEST KIT; and compatible when used as a TEST KIT.	A Human Immunodeficiency Virus (HIV) Enzyme Linked ImmunoSorbent Assay (ELISA) TEST KIT may contain controls, calibrators and washing buffers. All the reagents and articles are used together to detect HIV and therefore can be registered as a TEST KIT. These reagents and articles can be supplied separately as replacement items for that particular TEST KIT.

Table 2.12 **Continued**

Category	Description	Examples
SYSTEM	A number of constituent-components, that are: from the same product owner; intended to be used in combination to complete a common intended purpose; compatible when used as a SYSTEM; and sold under a single SYSTEM name or the labeling, IFU, brochures or catalogues for each constituent component states that the constituent component is intended for use with the SYSTEM.	A hip replacement SYSTEM comprising of femoral and acetabular components can be registered as a SYSTEM. The components must be used in combination to achieve a common intended purpose of total hip replacement. The size of the components may vary.
IVD CLUSTER	An IVD CLUSTER comprises of a number of *in vitro* diagnostic reagents or articles that are: from the same product owner; within risk classification A or B; of a common test methodology as listed in Annex 6 of GN-12; and of the same IVD CLUSTER category as listed in Annex 6 of GN-12.	
GROUP	A collection of two or more medical devices, supplied in a single package by a product owner. The medical device GROUP has the following: a single proprietary GROUP name, and a common intended purpose.	A first aid kit consisting of medical devices such as bandages, gauzes, drapes and thermometers, when assembled together as one package by a product owner, can be registered as a GROUP.

The content is accurate as of July 2015, please refer to HSA website for updated information.

2.9 Conclusions

The regulations for medical devices differ in the various markets, such as the classification and conformity systems. A manufacturer of medical devices always intends to sell the devices in multiple markets and must conform to systems where the device is marketed. But for the startups, the EU market is recommended instead of the US market due to the less complicated approval process and shorter duration.

FAQs

(1) What is the CE mark?

The letter *CE* stands for Conformité Européenne in French, which literally means "European Conformity." The CE mark is the proof from the manufacturer that the product is in conformity with the regulations. CE marking allows freedom of movement of the medical device in the territory of the European Union.

(2) What is a Competent Authority?

The list of Competent Authorities in the EU can be found at http://www.ema.europa.eu/ema/index.jsp?curl=pages/medicines/general/general_content_000155.jsp. Normally, each member state has one Competent Authority. But some countries have two, such as Poland, which has the Office for Registration of Medicinal Products, Medical Devices, and Biocidal Products and the Main Pharmaceutical Inspectorate.

(3) What is a notified body?

A notified body is a certification organization authorized by the relevant member state's competent authority to perform conformity assessment tasks specified in the directives. The notified body is responsible for evaluating the conformity of the product with the essential requirements and it issues the CE mark certificate.

(4) Can we be sure that a product affixed with the CE marking is safe?

Unfortunately, due to counterfeiting or misuse of the marking, there is never a 100% guarantee that a product bearing the CE marking is safe. However, with the adoption of Regulation 765/2008 and Decision 768/2008, the obligations of the manufacturer are spelled out and it is clear that by affixing the CE marking to a product, the manufacturer assumes full responsibility for its compliance with all applicable requirements in EU legislation.

It is the system behind the CE marking that ensures its proper functioning. The entire system, consisting of manufacturers, importers, distributors, notified bodies, and market surveillance authorities, has been strengthened through the New Legislative Framework, which aims to further reduce burdens on trade while, at the same time ensuring a high level of safety and protection of other public interests.

(5) How are medical devices classified?

Medical devices are classified by the level of risk.

(6) Will a medical device that has been categorized as Class II in China be categorized by the United States to be Class II?

The same category in different countries may not be equivalent to each other.

(7) What contributes to the risk level of a medical device?

The risk level is attributed by considering a series of factors, including the duration and type of the device's contact with the body; the degree of the invasiveness; whether the device requires surgery to implant it or if it can be used externally; and whether the device contains a component, which in its own right is considered to be a medicinal substance and has action ancillary to that of the device.

(8) Which of the following is higher in the hierarchy—Act, Regulation, or Standard?

Act is highest in the hierarchy, followed by Regulation, then Standard.

(9) How many devices were categorized under Class I?

There are about 780 device types under Class I and only about 50 device types require the 510(k).

(10) What is 510(k) and PMA?

510(k) is also known as premarket notification, and PMA is premarket approval.

(11) How do I know if my device requires a 510(k)?

To determine if a device requires a 510(k), a check with the FDA will be required. There are two methods for accomplishing this: go directly to the Classification database (http://www.accessdata.fda.gov/scripts/cdrh/cfdocs/cfpcd/classification.cfm) and search for a part of the device name, or, if you know the device panel (medical specialty to which your device belongs, go directly to the listing for that panel; http://www.fda.gov/MedicalDevices/DeviceRegulationandGuidance/Overview/ClassifyYourDevice/ucm051530.htm) and identify your device and the corresponding regulation.

(12) What are the Class I devices that are exempted from the GMP requirements with the exception of complaint files and general record keeping requirements?

Refer to the US Food and Drug Administration. (2014). Class I/II Exemptions. Retrieved from http://www.fda.gov/MedicalDevices/DeviceRegulationandGuidance/Overview/ClassifyYourDevice/ucm051549.htm.

(13) How is the public's health safeguarded after a device is on the market?

The public's safety is ensured through a series of postmarket surveillance activities, including adverse event reporting and continual postmarket studies to ascertain and monitor the device's safety and effectiveness.

(14) How are classifications and exemptions determined in the EU?

The panel in the EU that was assigned to the device determines the Class and other controls and exemptions.

(15) What is the process for marketing a device in the EU?

The general outline of the process to market a device in the EU is as follows: Choosing the appropriate directive, classification of the device, selection of the Notified Body, obtaining the conformity certification, affixing the CE mark, placing the device on the market, and reporting adverse events.

(16) Are State Food and Drug Administration (SFDA) and Chinese Food and Drug Administration (CFDA) the same? How are SFDA and CFDA related?

In March of 2013, SFDA was restructured from previous State Food and Drug Administration (SFDA) to the Chinese Food and Drug Administration (CFDA), which was announced in the decision made by the State Council.

(17) Our product licenses were issued by SFDA, are they still valid under the CFDA?

Unless otherwise stated, all the documents and decisions released by the SFDA retain validity for the CFDA.

Quality management systems for medical device manufacture

3

3.1 Introduction

To prevent fraudulent medical devices from entering the market, an effective quality management system is mandatory for medical device manufacturers before their products can enter the target market. The requirements vary in different countries according to their different regulations on medical devices. The two major regulations/standards for medical device manufacture are the ISO 13485 "Medical devices—Quality management systems: requirements for regulatory purposes," and the 21 CFR Parts 820 Quality Systems Regulations (USFDA). Most countries have adopted modified versions of the ISO 13485 and/or the USFDA regulations [54]. In the EU, ISO 13485 certification by a Notified Body (NB) could help the medical device manufacturers meet the compliance requirements of the EU directives, thus the manufacturers are allowed to market their medical devices within the European Union. However, ISO 13485 certification is not sufficient for the manufacturers who intend to sell medical devices in the United States; compliance with the Quality System Regulation (QSR) (21 CFR 820) is required.

A standard is an agreed upon, repeatable way of doing something. It is a document, published after collective work from one or more committees, which contains a technical specification or other precise criteria designed to be used consistently as a rule, guideline, or definition [55]. Standards have two main functions—ensuring the reliability and improving the effectiveness of goods and services. Standards are designed for voluntary use and do not impose any regulations. However, laws and regulations may refer to certain standards and make compliance with them compulsory. Based on the international standards ISO 13485, a lot of countries developed their own regulations for medical device manufacture, and a good understanding of ISO 13485 could facilitate the establishment of a quality management system for medical devices. In the United States, the QSR was published with the idea of international harmonization with international standards in mind; the ISO 13485 is not identical to QSR in the United States.

Following the regulations mentioned in Chapter 2, the two main quality management systems for medical device manufacture introduced in this chapter are ISO 13485 and 21 CFR 820.

Medical devices. http://dx.doi.org/10.1016/B978-0-08-100289-6.00003-X

3.1.1 History of QSR 21 CFR 820

Consumers expect all medical devices they use to meet quality standards. To achieve consistently satisfactory quality, the medical devices production process must be strictly controlled to ensure the safety and effectiveness of the devices. The QSR 21 CFR 820 and ISO 13485 are two main systems applicable globally to ensuring that the medical device manufacture processes are safe and effective.

According to an FDA report released in September 1970, around 10,000 injuries and 731 deaths were caused by ineffective medical devices [54]. The report provided information that made it clear that there was a necessity to form a regulatory system and body. The requirements for records and reports; registration and inspection of establishments; and uniform quality assurance programs were proposed, and it was called good manufacturing practices (GMP), all these were established and went into effect on December 18, 1978. On November 28, 1990, the FDA was authorized to add preproduction design controls to the GMP regulation. Since then, strict controls of the design and development processes were required for medical device manufacturers. The regulation also incorporated a provision to include the oversight of foreign countries selling products in the United States—QSR 21 CFR parts 820 was then drafted. Efforts were made to harmonize this regulation with both the ISO 9001 (Quality management systems—Requirements) and ISO 13485 (Medical devices—Quality management systems—Requirements for regulatory purposes). The regulations are a framework for manufacturers and provide sufficient flexibility for them to formulate and implement those parts of the regulation that are applicable to their products, processes, and the risk of their products [56–58]. The 21 CFR 820 was first published in 1997, and is also called current good manufacturing practice (cGMP) [59, 60]. The brief description of the GMP evolution is shown in the left section of Figure 3.1.

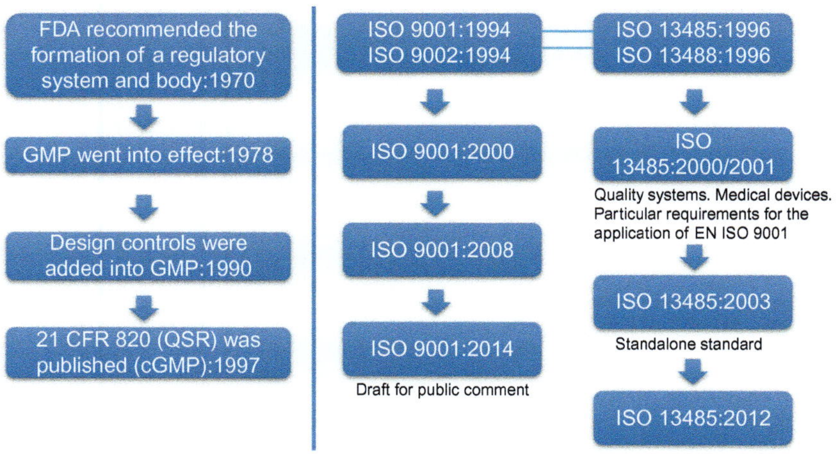

Figure 3.1 The evolution of ISO 13485:2012 and QSR.

3.1.2 History of ISO 13485

ISO 13485:1996 was published by the ISO technical committee 210 Working Group 1, following alignment with ISO 9001:1994. ISO 13485:1996 made reference to ISO 9001 throughout, and as such was not a standalone standard [55]. In 2000, the Standard EN ISO 13485:1996 and EN ISO 13488:1996 were accepted as European Standards for replacing the EN 46001 and the EN 46002. These standards were published as EN ISO 13485:2000 and EN ISO 13488:2000. ISO also published ISO 13485:2001. Actually, ISO 13485:2001 is identical to ISO 13485:2000 and ISO 13485:1996. ISO 13485:2003 was a standalone standard, and currently it has been replaced by ISO 13485:2012. Actually, ISO 13485:2003 and ISO 13485:2012 are identical in terms of the requirements except that ISO13485:2012 includes Annexes which specify where clauses of the ISO 13485 covers the EU directive requirements. The evolution of ISO 13485 is shown in Figure 3.1 on the right side.

3.2 ISO 13485:2012

3.2.1 General requirements of ISO 13485: 2012

ISO 13485:2012 [4] specifies requirements for a quality management system where an organization needs to demonstrate its ability to provide medical devices and related services that consistently meet applicable customer and regulatory requirements. The primary objective of this international standard is to facilitate harmonized medical device regulatory requirements for quality management systems.

ISO 13485 is harmonized with ISO 9001, with some differences. As a result, it includes some particular requirements for medical devices and excludes some of the regulatory requirements of ISO 9001:2000 that are not appropriate as regulatory requirements.

The ISO 13485 standard has eight sections, three of them are general information for manufacturers about the standard and not auditable. Certification focuses on the five key auditable sections [61]:

(1) the quality management system;
(2) management responsibility;
(3) resource management;
(4) product realization; and
(5) measurement, analysis, and improvement.

Figure 3.2 summarizes the process required by ISO 13485:2012, namely, establishment, implementation, and maintenance, and emphasizes the importance of documentation, including a quality manual, control of records, and documents.

3.2.2 Document control required by ISO 13485:2012

The requirements for documents and records are specified in Section 3.2.4.2 of ISO 13485, and it has been divided into four tiers with their own types of documentation (Table 3.1).

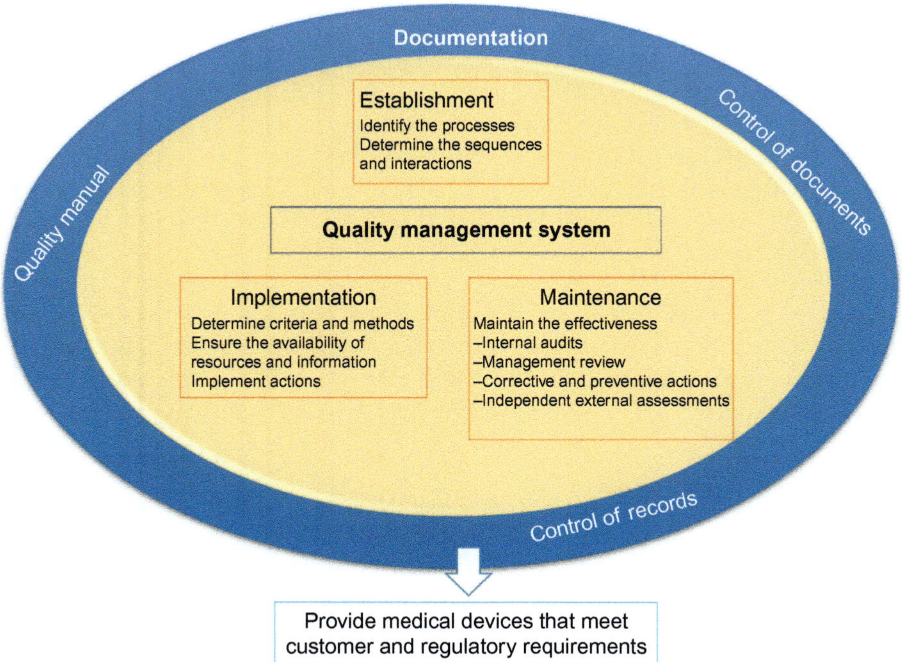

Figure 3.2 The general requirements of ISO 13485.

Table 3.1 Four-tier quality management setup

Level	Documents	Descriptions
1	Quality manual	Description of the QMS in accordance with policy and objectives
2	Quality procedures	Interrelated processes and activities (who, what, why, when, where)
3	Work instructions and other documents needed to plan, operate, and control processes where required	Detailed work documents (how)
4	Evidence of results achieved and activities performed	Records

3.2.2.1 Quality manual

A quality manual is unique to each organization. A small organization may find it appropriate to include the description of its entire quality management system within a single manual, including all the documented procedures required by ISO 13485.

Large, multinational organizations may need several manuals at the global, national, or regional level, and a more complex hierarchy of documentation.

A quality manual is the top-level document defining the following elements, but not necessarily in the same order:

(1) Title and scope;
(2) Tables of content;
(3) Review, approval, and revision;
(4) Quality policy and objectives;
(5) Organization, responsibility, and authority;
(6) References;
(7) Quality management system description; and
(8) Appendices [62].

Additional information relating to quality manuals is available in ISO/TR 10013: Guidelines for quality management system documentation [62]. Template documentation of a quality manual that meets the requirements of ISO 13485 can be accessed online [63].

3.2.2.2 Control of documents

Documents could be: plans, requirements, or specifications for realization or activities; input for a process; communication of information; or sharing of knowledge, information, or data [64].

The documentation system must cover all new documents and changes to existing controlled documents, and the following aspects must be ensured [65]:

(1) Accuracy and use of documents are controlled;
(2) Obsolete documents are removed or prevented from being used;
(3) All documentation is adequate for its purpose.

3.2.2.3 Control of records

Records could be: those papers related to the design and the manufacturing process, affecting all medical devices of a particular type; those that relate to the manufacture or distribution of an individual medical device or batch of medical devices; or those that demonstrate the effective operation of the overall quality management system. Records should be maintained by all personnel performing the task, operation, or activity, results of which need to be recorded. The following aspects must be taken into consideration for control of records [66,67]:

(1) Records are used to prove that requirements have been met;
(2) A controlled procedure to manage medical device records needs to be developed;
(3) Electronic records should be regularly backed up;
(4) Records related to medical devices should be retained;
(5) The quality system is operated in accordance with documented procedures that must be effective.

Quality records are important, especially in ISO 13485, as they are the evidence that activities that are required as part of the quality management system have been completed. Requirements for records are referenced in at least 50 places within the standard [55].

3.2.3 Processes required by ISO 13485

3.2.3.1 Implementation

For implementation of ISO 13485:2012, a company can follow the process as [68,69] shown in Figure 3.3:

(1) Define quality policy;
(2) Define scope;
(3) Identify regulations and requirements;
(4) Train, implement, measure, and sustain;
(5) Select procedures, records, objectives, and controls to be implemented;
(6) Review policies and procedures in place;
(7) Internal audit;
(8) Complete and get ISO 13485 certification.

The processes for product realization are the basis of a quality management system (QMS). It is suggested to draw a general flowchart of the process, describing how the product will be realized. The process should be:

(1) Receiving an order;
(2) Scheduling;
(3) Purchasing raw materials;
(4) Production;
(5) Packaging; and
(6) Delivery.

According to the main process, subprocesses derived will be included under the quality management system. Subprocesses can be defined according to the products.

Another way to implement would be to divide activity into different areas according to the standard suggestions and identify which processes are related in each area [64]:

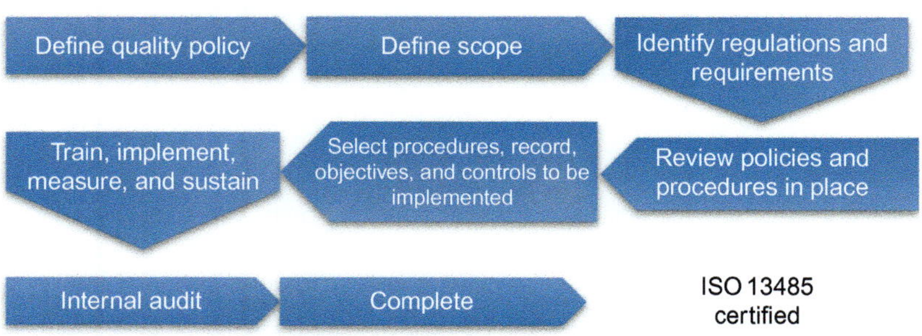

Figure 3.3 Steps to getting ISO 13485 certified.

(1) Work environment;
(2) Review of requirements related to the product;
(3) Validation of processes;
(4) Preservation of property; and
(5) Control of purchasing.

3.2.3.2 Process effectiveness

Effectiveness is the extent to which planned activities are realized and planned results achieved. The ISO 13485 requires constant maintenance of the effectiveness of the quality management system (while ISO 9001 requires continual improvement of the effectiveness).

Ways to maintain the effectiveness of the quality management system are [70]:

(1) Internal audits (the audit evaluates whether the activities are performed and how well they are performed);
(2) Management review;
(3) Corrective and preventive actions; and
(4) Independent external assessments.

And following are some examples:

(1) Defining and promoting processes which lead to achieving regulatory compliance;
(2) Acquiring and using process data and information on a continuing basis;
(3) Determining and providing resources, including human and information system resources;
(4) Directing necessary changes to the quality management system; and
(5) Using suitable evaluation methods such as internal audits and management reviews.

Maintaining the effectiveness of the quality management system in its ability to meet customer and regulatory requirements will typically involve the organization responding effectively to external factors, such as:

(1) Changes in regulatory requirements, including adverse event reporting and
(2) Customer feedback.

And internal changes, such as changes to

(1) Key personnel;
(2) Facilities;
(3) Manufacturing processes and equipment, including related software;
(4) Software related to the quality management system; and
(5) Product, including software.

3.2.4 Conformity assessment, registration, and certification processes

3.2.4.1 Conformity assessment

The use of harmonized standards is an integral part of conformity assessment. Devices of different classifications are subjected to different "conformity assessment reviews."

The detail and complexity of the procedures vary according to the potential risk of the device [71].

Conformity assessment is the process used to show that a product, service, or system meets specified requirements. These requirements are likely to be contained in an ISO standard. But an ISO itself does not perform conformity assessments. In the EU, the conformity assessment can be done by a third-party NB.

Conducting and being qualified for a conformity assessment have a number of benefits, such as it could provide consumers with added confidence and give the company a competitive edge.

The main forms of conformity assessment are certification, inspection, and testing. Certification is the provision by an independent body of written assurance that the product, service, or system in question meets specific requirements. Certification is also known as third-party conformity assessment. Inspection describes the regular checking of a product to make sure it meets specified criteria. Testing is the determination of one or more of an object's or product's characteristics and is usually performed by a laboratory.

Market introduction of medical devices is preceded by certification and registration, which are accomplished in compliance with national and international regulations. For example, certification by placing the CE-mark is a requirement for selling most medical products and equipment in the EU. For certification, each country has appointed one or more authorities to perform the certification procedure. In Europe, these authorities are named NBs and operate independently of each other. The objective of a NBs is to assess the performance of medical devices in terms of performance and safety, while evidence of effectiveness is not required at the stage of certification.

For example, a conformity assessment procedure in the European Union demonstrates that the device complies with the requirements of Directive 93/42/EEC. Compliance is stated by establishing a Conformity Declaration. The classification of the device dictates the appropriate conformity assessment procedure. In some cases the manufacturer has a choice of conformity routes [72].

3.2.4.2 Certification

Formal certification is achieved only through external (third party) assessment by a Certification Body. ISO 13485 certification could help a medical device company obtain expanded access to the world market and improved ability to bid for contracts.

The display of the certification mark (a symbol granted by the certification body which usually is a combination of the registrar's logo and ISO 13485) and the evidence of independent audits by professional, independent certification bodies designated by an accreditation agency can help to provide a much greater trust in the company's ability to provide a consistent high quality product or service.

Medical device manufacturers who wish to obtain ISO 13485 certification need to educate themselves on the requirements of regulators and customers, as well as on what an ISO 13485 compliant management system will entail.

(1) The first step to create the management system should be drafting a quality manual; the quality manual should outline the organization's goals, processes, and procedures for compliance and quality management.
   - An employee with the know-how to develop and implement such a program can help create the management system.
   - A consultant with an expertise in the ISO 13485 market can be hired.

(2) Seeking a certification body
   - The registrar is accredited by an accrediting body to award ISO 13485 certification.
   - Keep the target market in mind. For instance, if a medical device manufacturer wants to sell in North America, it should seek certification through a registrar accredited by a North American accreditation body to ensure they will meet country-specific or customer requirements.

(3) After certification, an organization will be subjected to on-going surveillance by its certification body. The duration of the assessment is contingent on an organization's scope—its size, number of personnel, and type and complexity of products manufactured. The frequency of surveillance assessments will be determined by an organization's scope as well as its performance, though they will usually be conducted annually or semi-annually. However, organizations should expect a complete reassessment 3 years after initial certification.

3.2.5 ISO 13485 application in various countries

ISO 13485 is the most commonly chosen path for companies to meet the QMS requirements in Europe, Canada, Japan, Australia, and other countries [73]. But there might be slight differences when a manufacturer intends to meet the requirements of the QSR in different countries, and this is highlighted in the following.

3.2.5.1 EU

EN ISO 13485:2012 has been harmonized with the three EU Medical Devices directives (the details can be found in Chapter 2), so certification to this standard by an accredited certification body automatically presumes compliance with specific clauses in these directives [74].

3.2.5.2 Canada

Medical device manufacturers who want to access the Canadian market must, as part of the requirements to obtain and maintain a medical device license from Health Canada, be registered in accordance to ISO 13485 under the requirements of a Canadian Medical Devices Conformity Assessment System (CMDCAS) recognized registrar.

3.2.5.3 Japan

Japan's MHLW issued Ministerial Ordinance #169 describing the quality management system requirements for medical devices. As part of the Japanese registration process for medical devices, a QMS conformity assessment is required. Japan has largely embraced ISO 13485 as the basis for their QMS requirements. Manufacturers with ISO 13485 in place will easily meet Ministerial Ordinance #169 by adjusting some gaps between ISO 13485 and Ordinance #169 [75].

MHLW Ministerial Ordinance #169 is very similar to ISO 13485, but it has some additional requirements such as [76]:

(1) Additional requirements regarding infrastructure;
(2) Written procedures of training; and
(3) A retention period of obsolete controlled documents and records.

In summary, companies should also take note of the following aspects of ISO 13485 standards:

(1) ISO 13485 was written as a model to meet the quality system requirements of various global regulations; if a company meets ISO 13485 requirements, it should easily be able to meet the FDA QSR requirements. Although ISO 13485 has not been adopted by the FDA, the FDA participated in writing ISO 13485 to ensure the requirements are aligned.
(2) Risk management is a key element of ISO 13485, and ISO 14971 [77] serves as a guide for risk management.
(3) TR 14969 [78] is a guidance document for the use and implementation of ISO 13485.
(4) Companies considering ISO 13485 certification need to understand the regulatory requirements of the countries in which their products are to be sold, and choose a service provider that is recognized in the market they intend to enter. For example, only certificates accredited under the CMDCAS by the Standards Council of Canada will be recognized by Health Canada in applying for a medical device license. For an EU member country, the service provider must be a NB.

3.3 Current good manufacturing practice

The quality systems for FDA-regulated products (food, drugs, biologics, and devices) are known as cGMPs. The cGMP requirements for medical devices in part 820 (21 CFR part 820) were first authorized by section 520(f) of the Federal Food, Drug, and Cosmetic Act (the act) (21 U.S.C. 360j(f)), which was among the authorities added to the act by the Medical Device Amendments of 1976 (Pub. L. 94–295) [57]. The cGMP provides systems that assure proper design, monitoring, and control of manufacturing processes and facilities. Compliance with the cGMP regulations assures the identity, strength, quality, and purity of medical devices by requiring that manufacturers of medical devices adequately control manufacturing operations. This includes establishing strong quality management systems, obtaining appropriate quality raw materials, establishing robust operating procedures, detecting and investigating product quality deviations, and maintaining reliable testing laboratories. This formal system will help to prevent instances of contamination, mix-ups, deviations, failures, and errors. This assures that medical device products meet their quality standards.

The cGMP requirements are flexible enough to allow each manufacturer to decide individually how to best implement the necessary controls by using scientifically sound designs, processing methods, and testing procedures. The flexibility allows and encourages companies to use modern technologies and innovative approaches to achieve higher quality through continual improvement. Accordingly, the "c" in cGMP stand for "current," requiring companies to use technologies and systems that

Table 3.2 **Compliance requirements for QSR**

Manufacture place	Marketing place	Compliance with QSR
US	US	Required
US	Outside US	Not required
Outside US	US	Required
Outside US	Outside US	Not required

are up to date in order to comply with regulations. Systems and equipment that may have been "top-of-the-line" in preventing contamination, mix-ups, and errors 10 or 20 years ago may be less than adequate by today's standards [79].

The cGMPs are minimum requirements, and many medical device manufacturers have already implemented comprehensive and advanced quality systems and risk management approaches that far exceed these minimum standards. The QSR system contains seven subsystems: managements, design control, corrective and preventive actions, production and process controls, facility and equipment controls, materials controls, and record/documents/change controls [80].

Suppliers of raw materials or components do not have to comply with the regulations, but they are subject to the purchasing controls of the regulations. Medical device manufacturers must establish procedures and controls with their suppliers for essential raw materials that include quality metrics, material performance and purity specifications, assurance of supply, and notification of any formulation or process changes.

It is important to note that compliance requirements for QSR is subjected to the marketplace within or outside the United States [81]. If a manufacturer would like to market its medical device in the United States, compliance with the QSR is mandatory (shown in Table 3.2).

3.4 The difference between ISO 13485 and cGMP

ISO 13485 is required in Europe, Canada, and many other countries for medical devices. In the United States, the FDA QSR is required. Although the QSR is structured very differently than ISO 13485, they have no conflicting requirements.

In ISO 13485, meeting requirements includes meeting regulatory requirements. So for devices that will be used in the United States, to be compliant with ISO 13485, manufacturers must also meet the QSR. As a regulation, the QSR is more specific than ISO 13485, particularly in the areas of training, design controls, complaint handling, labeling control, document and change controls, and production and process controls [80,82]. The USFDA also does not require a quality manual, unlike ISO 13485 (Table 3.3).

While being certified to ISO 13485 does not fulfill the requirements of either the USFDA or other regulators, the certification aligns an organization's management system to the requirements of the USFDA's QSR requirements as well as many other

Table 3.3 Comparison between ISO 13485 and 21 CFR 820

ISO 13485	21 CFR 820 (cGMP)
4 Quality management system	Subpart B Quality system requirements
4.1 General requirements	Section 820.20 Management responsibility
4.2 Documentation requirements	Section 820.22 Quality audit
5 Management responsibility	Section 820.25 Personnel
5.1 Management commitment	Subpart C Design controls
5.2 Customer focus	Section 820.30 Design controls
5.3 Quality policy	Subpart D Document controls
5.4 Planning	Section 820.40 Document controls
5.5 Responsibility, authority and communication	Subpart E Purchasing controls
5.6 Management review	Section 820.50 Purchasing controls
6 Resource management	Subpart F Identification and traceability
6.1 Provision of resources	Section 820.60 Identification
6.2 Human resources	Section 820.65 Traceability
6.3 Infrastructure	Subpart G Production and process controls
6.4 Work environment	Section 820.70 Production and process controls
7 Product realization	Section 820.72 Inspection, measuring, and test equipment
7.1 Planning of product realization	Section 820.75 Process validation
7.2 Customer-related processes	Subpart H Acceptance activities
7.3 Design and development	Section 820.86 Acceptance status
7.4 Purchasing	Subpart I Nonconforming product
7.5 Production and service provision	Section 829.90 Nonconforming product
7.6 Control of monitoring and measuring devices	Subpart J Corrective and preventive action
8 Measurement, analysis and improvement	Section 820.100 Corrective and preventive action
8.1 General	Subpart K Labeling and packaging control
8.2 Monitoring and measurement	Section 820.120 Device labeling
8.3 Control of nonconforming product	Section 820.130 Device packaging
8.4 Analysis of data	Section 820.140 Handling
8.5 Improvement	Subpart L Handling, storage, distribution and installation
	Section 820.150 Storage
	Section 820.160 Distribution
	Section 820.170 Installation
	Subpart M Records
	Section 820.180 General requirements
	Section 820.181 Device master record

Table 3.3 Continued

ISO 13485	21 CFR 820 (cGMP)
	Section 820.184 Device history record Section 820.186 Quality system record Section 820.198 Complaint files Subpart N Servicing Section 820.200 Servicing Subpart O Statistical techniques Section 820.250 Statistical techniques

regulatory requirements found throughout the world. Therefore, ISO 13485 certification serves to create a management system that can be thought of as a framework on which to build compliance to various regulatory and customer requirements.

3.5 Conclusions

The medical device market has become globalized, the industry and the regulatory authorities across the world have been drawn closer together. Though ISO 13485 certification is not mandatory in most markets, it is still very helpful for companies to achieve the certification in terms of:

(1) Increased efficiency, better product quality, and improved customer service;
(2) Ease of access to new markets: the certification is recognized by many governments, and may satisfy some or all of the quality system requirements in multiple countries.

In today's globalized world, the need for regulatory harmonization is greater than ever, particularly in the growing and highly regulated medical industry. Achieving ISO 13485 certification will help manufacturers of medical devices and providers of medical services compete today—and may prove absolutely crucial in the future [83]. ISO 13485 certification is a stepping stone to securing and maintaining global business.

FAQs

(1) What is the relationship between cGMP, QSR, and 21 CFR 820?
The current good manufacturing practices (cGMP) requirements set forth in the Quality System Regulation (QSR) was promulgated under section 520 of the Food, Drug, and Cosmetic (FD&C) Act. And the QSR is in Part 820 of Title 21 of the Code of Federal Regulations (21 CFR 820). So, in this book, cGMP, QSR, and 21 CFR 820 are almost equivalent to each other.

(2) Who can be certified to ISO 13485?
If an organization designs or manufactures medical devices, raw materials, or provides services related to medical devices, such as sterilization, installation, labeling, or technical publication, it can be certified to ISO 13485.

(3) Must a medical device manufacturer become ISO 13485 certified?

Part of the answer lies in what is required by the regulatory agencies of the countries in which devices are sold. For certain types of devices, companies must have their quality management system certified to ISO 13485 to legally sell or market devices in Canada and the countries of the European Union, for example. It also help companies in obtaining the product certification CE mark for their devices.

(4) Why are cGMPs so important?

Compliance with cGMPs ensures that facilities are in good condition; equipment is properly maintained and calibrated; employees are qualified and fully trained; processes are reliable and reproducible; and, finally, it assures the quality of medical devices.

(5) What is the difference between ISO 13485:2003 and ISO 13485:2012?

EN ISO 13485:2012 is the same as ISO 13485:2003 in terms of the requirements except that for EN ISO 13485:2012, it includes Annexes which specify where clauses of the ISO 13485 covers the EU directive requirements. It is important to note that the text of the global standard ISO 13485:2003 is unchanged. Only the foreword and annexes in the European version have been revised.

(6) What is the difference between ISO 9001 and ISO 13485?

Though based on ISO 9001, ISO 13485 removes 9001's emphasis on continual improvement and customer satisfaction. In its place is an emphasis on meeting regulatory as well as customer requirements, risk management, and maintaining effective processes, namely, the process specific to the safe design, manufacture, and distribution of medical devices. The purpose of ISO 13485 certification is sometimes misunderstood. ISO 13485 certification does not fulfill the requirements of 9001, nor is it equivalent to, or have the ability to take the place of, any country-specific requirement for medical device manufacture. The standard is, in part, meant to serve as a means to the creation of a management system that aligns with the requirements of various regulators.

(7) Is ISO 13485 certification sufficient for the manufacturers who intend to sell medical devices in the United States? If not, what other requirements are needed?

No. Additional compliance with the Quality System Regulation (21 CFR 820) is required.

(8) What are the auditable sections for ISO 13485?

There are five sections that are auditable for ISO 13485. They are the quality management system, management responsibility, resource management, product realization, and the last section would be measurement, analysis, and improvement.

(9) What are the documentations required by ISO 13485:2012?

Refer to Table 3.1. Four-tier quality management system setup for a brief guide.

(10) Are there any examples of documentation of a quality manual to meet the requirements of ISO 13485?

Template documentation of a quality manual that meets the requirements of ISO 13485 can be accessed online at http://www.isoxp.com/10Products/ISO13485Docu.aspx.

(11) Why are quality records so important?

Quality records are important because they are evidence that activities that are required as part of the quality management system have been completed. Requirements for records are referenced in at least 50 places within the ISO 13485 standard.

(12) What are the steps to getting ISO 13485 certification?

The steps are as follow: define quality policy; define scope; identify regulation and requirements; review policies and procedures in place; select procedures; record objectives and controls to be implemented; train, implement, measure, and sustain; internal audit; and, finally, upon completion, get ISO 13485 certified.

(13) Can subprocess be excluded from the QMS?

According to the main process, subprocesses derived will be included under the quality management system.

(14) How are ISO 13485 and ISO 9001 different?

ISO 13485 requires constant maintenance of the effectiveness of the quality management system, while ISO 9001 requires continual improvement of the effectiveness.

(15) What are some of the ways to maintain the effectiveness of the quality management system?

Internal audits, management reviews, and corrective and preventive actions as well as independent external assessments. For more information, please refer to ISO 14969:2005—Guidance on the application of ISO 13485:2003.

(16) What are the benefits of being qualified for a conformity assessment?

It provides the consumer with added confidence and gives the company a more competitive edge in the market.

(17) Do the different Notified Bodies issue the same certification? Are they based on identical standards?

Yes, they are all based on the same standard set by the EU regulatory authority.

(18) Is Certification Body the same as Notified Body?

These terms are often used interchangeably to describe third-party organizations that conduct certification audits of medical device companies to ensure compliance with the ISO 13485 Standard and associated Directives. The difference between them is the scope of their auditing authority by geographic market.

The process of gaining approval for new medical devices

4

4.1 Introduction

In Chapters 2 and 3 we covered the regulatory framework for various countries and quality management systems. The regulatory framework provides the basis of how each country monitors and controls the design, manufacture, and marketing of medical devices. The most crucial part of these processes is to ensure the safety and effectiveness of a device during the manufacturing process. And thus, quality management systems are set in place to reinforce and control the entire manufacturing process. While making sure that requirements for these processes are met, regulatory bodies do require documents, certifications, and so on to verify that each step is appropriately controlled and maintained. The steps for gaining approval (Figure 4.1) and documents required for submission will be covered in this chapter.

Using the USFDA as an example, one must have a basic understanding that all medical devices are subjected to General Controls and they must conform to cGMPs covered under 21 CFR 820—Quality System Regulation (QSR). However, do note that there are a handful of Class I devices that are exempted from GMP requirements. In terms of regulation, the USFDA is considered the most comprehensive and stringent of all, and thus, will be covered in more depth. Procedures and documents for the EU, China, and Singapore will be briefly covered in this chapter as well.

4.2 The United States

In this subsection, we focus on the steps to market a device and the preparation of a dossier for premarket notification (PMN) 510(k) and premarket approval (PMA) submission in the United States. The 510(k), otherwise known as PMN, is unique to the FDA and its clearance permits manufacturers to market their device on the basis that the device to be marketed is as safe and effective as another previously legally marketed device. PMA is a more stringent premarket submission process, which requires clinical evidence to prove the safety and effectiveness of the device to be marketed.

The five general steps in Figure 4.1 for marketing a medical device are further expanded with respect to the USFDA regulations. The 510(k) notification and PMA approval are the means by which the USFDA regulates the safety and effectiveness of medical devices, thereby ensuring overall public health. The steps move from classification of a medical device and how to choose the appropriate premarket submission, to the actual documents and elements required in a premarket submission. Following that, we will briefly cover the USFDA review process and timeline, as well as establishment registration and device listing.

Medical devices. http://dx.doi.org/10.1016/B978-0-08-100289-6.00004-1

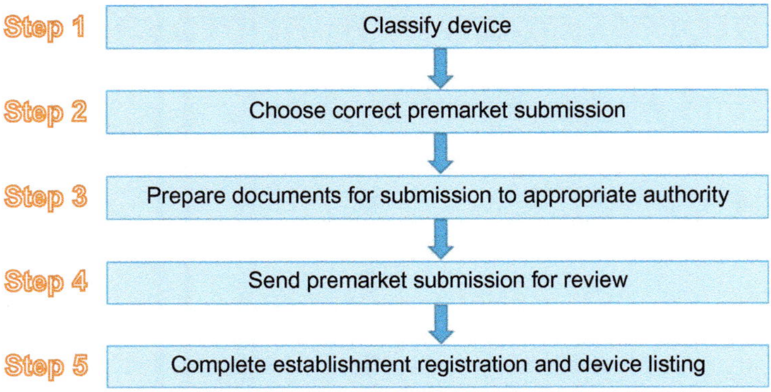

Figure 4.1 Steps to market your device.

4.2.1 Step 1: Classify device

Figure 4.2 describes the basic steps for FDA clearance (for 510[k]) or approval (in the case of PMA) before marketing a device. Step 1 refers to classification of the device, which was intensively covered in Chapter 2, where the risk level of the medical devices correlates with their assigned class as seen in Figure 2.3. The classification of a medical device is also dependent on its intended use. There are two ways to identify the class under which a device is classified.

Method 1: Using the FDA Product Classification Database (Figure 4.3) to find the product or predicate medical device, which has similar functionality to the medical

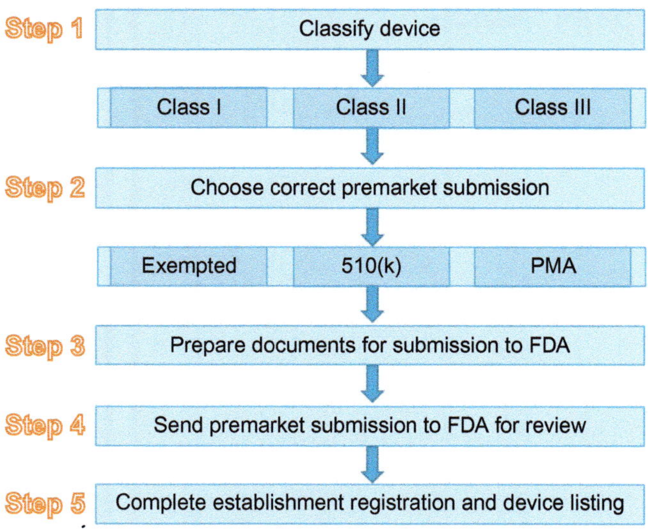

Figure 4.2 FDA premarket submission process in the United States.

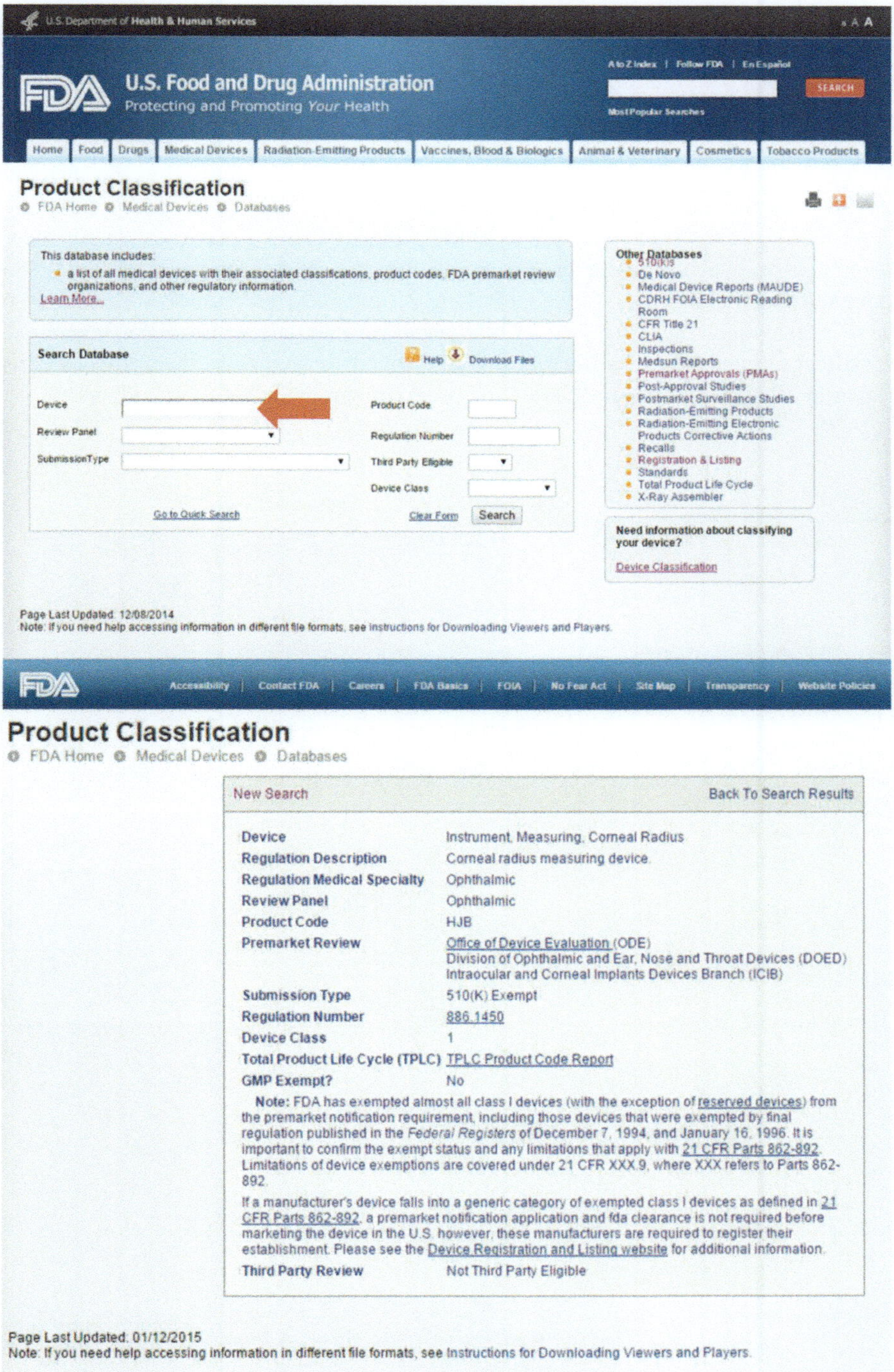

Figure 4.3 FDA Product Classification Database [84].

device, the class may be identified. Using a corneal radium measuring device as an example, type in a search under "Device" as shown in Figure 4.3, and the search result would show all information available such as the Product Code, Regulation Number, Device Class, etc.

Method 2: This method requires the use of the Medical Specialty Panels (Figure 4.4) to find the class of the medical device. After identifying the medical specialty of the device, the regulation citation (21 CFR) part number may be identified; using the same example as in the previous method, a corneal radius measuring device, which is an eye-care related device, would fall under 21 CFR Part 886 (Ophthalmic), and referring to the CFR Title 21, one may narrow down the search to the section number, e.g., 21 CFR 886.1450, where a short description of the device, the classification, and other information may be found. In this case, the corneal radius measuring device is a Class I device that is exempted from PMN procedures.

	Medical Specialty	Regulation Citation (21CFR)
73	Anesthesiology	Part 868
74	Cardiovascular	Part 870
75	Chemistry	Part 862
76	Dental	Part 872
77	Ear, Nose, and Throat	Part 874
78	Gastroenterology and Urology	Part 876
79	General and Plastic Surgery	Part 878
80	General Hospital	Part 880
81	Hematology	Part 864
82	Immunology	Part 866
83	Microbiology	Part 866
84	Neurology	Part 882
85	Obstetrical and Gynecological	Part 884
86	Ophthalmic	Part 886
87	Orthopedic	Part 888
88	Pathology	Part 864
89	Physical Medicine	Part 890
90	Radiology	Part 892
91	Toxicology	Part 862

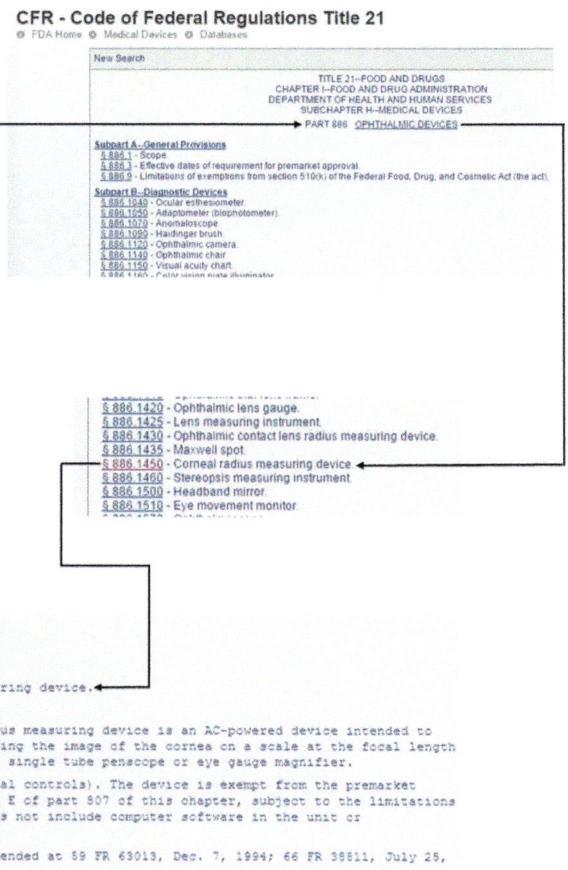

Figure 4.4 Medical Specialty Panel and 21 CFR 886.1450 [85].

4.2.2 Step 2: Choose correct premarket submission

Choosing correct premarket submission in Step 2 (Figure 4.2) may refer to either 510(k) or PMA, whichever the medical device classification specifies in the CFR. Class I and II medical devices are not as crucial to human life sustaining as Class III medical devices and hence, only require "clearance" for 510(k) before marketing or an exemption if stated in the CFR. For the latter, it requires more stringent controls and PMA "approval" before marketing. There are many types of submission as shown in Figure 4.5.

The FDA developed a guidance document in March 1998 called, "The New 510(k) Paradigm – Alternate Approaches to Demonstrating Substantial Equivalence in Premarket Notifications" (Figure 4.6) in order to make the PMN review process more efficient and provides two other alternatives to the original Traditional 510(k) submission; Special and Abbreviated 510(k). "The New 510(k) Paradigm" guidance also helps in the decision making process for choosing the right 510(k) submission method for a desired purpose by providing questions to direct submitters to the right method (Figure 4.6) [86].

Traditional 510(k) is the original complete submission as provided in the 21 CFR 807 and may be used for any type of 510(k) submission.

Special 510(k) submission is used for device modification of a company's own medical device that has previously been cleared under the 510(k) process. It is also used when the device design complies with the QSR Design Controls (21 CFR 820.30) and allows manufacturers to declare conformance to design controls without providing the data.

The abbreviated 510(k) submission method may be used when a guidance document exists, a special control has been established, or when the FDA has recognized a relevant consensus standard.

These 510(k) submission methods and contents will be discussed further in Section 4.2.3.2.2.

The *de novo* submission method is for novel medical devices that are of low to moderate risk (Class I and II), but have been classified automatically as Class III (high

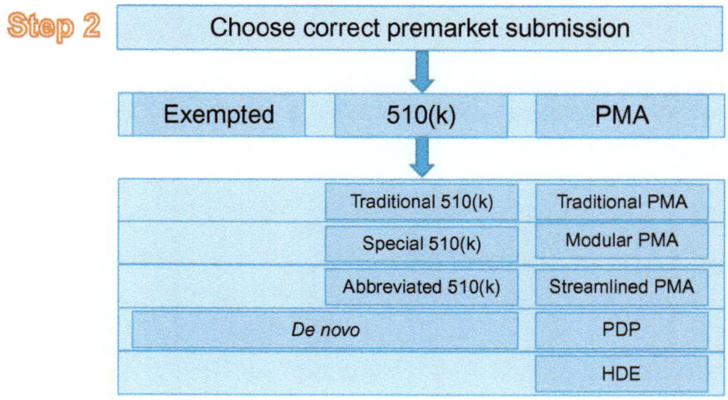

Figure 4.5 Premarket submission methods.

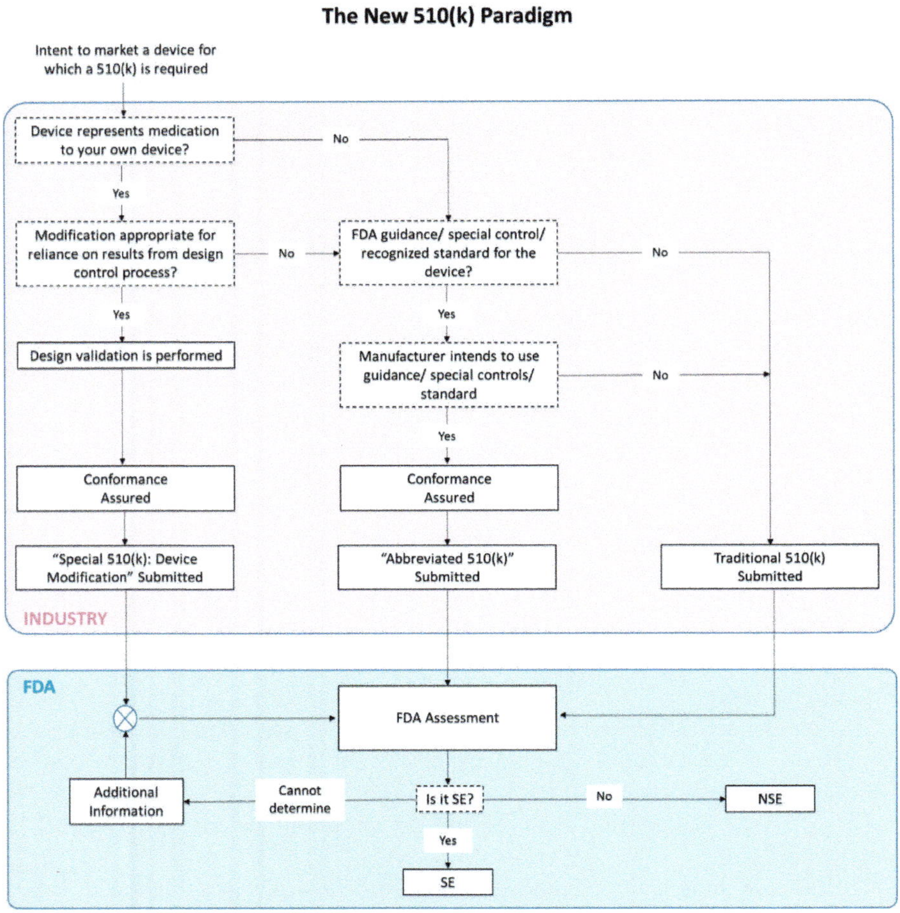

Figure 4.6 The New 510(k) Paradigm [86].

risk) devices because they do not have any legally marketed predicate device for comparison. It is also used when a 510(k) submission is deemed as nonsubstantial equivalence (NSE). A *de novo* submission to the FDA must then be made within 30 days upon receipt of the NSE determination, to request a risk-based evaluation for classification of the device into Class I or II [87].

There are a few types of PMA applications for more stringent controls as well as flexibility [88].

Traditional PMA is the original complete application whereby all the supporting documents, information, clinical studies, etc. are submitted to the FDA together in volumes. This method is used when clinical testing of the devices has been done in a country with established medical device regulation and the device has gained approval.

Modular PMA allows an application to be submitted in modules (well-delineated components) to the FDA, and eventually a complete PMA is compiled over a specified time period. This method is suitable for devices that are in the early stages of clinical study, but not suitable for those devices that are still in the design stage with likely alterations, as well as those on the verge of PMA submission.

Streamlined PMA is for a device that is well known to the FDA, that is, the FDA would have had many previous dealings with it, or for which an FDA guidance document or published methods for review have been evaluated by the FDA. Thus, the PMA submitted will be streamlined with a more efficient review process with the FDA's prior knowledge of the device.

For devices in early stages of design and development, the Product Development Protocol (PDP) method may be used. This method allows early interaction with the FDA to address FDA concerns and to come to an agreement on methods to prove the safety and effectiveness of a new device during its development stage. Upon FDA agreement to device details of design, development, its output, and acceptance criteria of outputs, the sponsor can provide the FDA important information as it is generated throughout the development process at certain milestones. A PDP is considered an approved PMA when the FDA declares a PDP completed.

A Humanitarian Device Exemption (HDE) application is submitted to the FDA to gain PMA for a Humanitarian Use Device (HUD), which is a device that is intended to treat or diagnose a medical condition that affects less than 4000 persons in the United States per year. The HDE application is similar to a normal PMA application, except that an HDE is not required to have scientifically valid clinical investigation results. However, it does require sufficient evidence to prove that the device does not pose significant risk and that the probable health benefits outweigh the risks involved. Furthermore, absence of a comparable device to treat the same condition must be established, otherwise, the device may not be marketed.

4.2.3 Step 3: Prepare documents for submission to the FDA

Preparation of a dossier for FDA submission can be a tedious process. However, with the understanding that all the information FDA requires is to ultimately establish that the device is safe and effective for use, the preparation of the dossier then becomes a logical process.

4.2.3.1 Class I process

Class I (low risk) medical devices are usually exempted from 510(k) or PMA and can be marketed immediately, unless otherwise stated in the CFR. They are all subjected to General Controls and current Good Manufacturing Practice (cGMP), however, a few of the devices are exempted from cGMP as well. For those that require 510 (k), please refer to Section 4.2.3.2.

4.2.3.2 Class II process—510(k)

Premarket notification, or 510(k), is submitted to the FDA to prove that the device to be marketed is substantially equivalent (SE) to a previously legally marketed device, also known as a predicate device. According to the FDA, a device is SE if, compared to a predicate, it has the:

- Same intended use; and
- Same technological characteristics;

  or
- Same intended use; and
- Different technological characteristics and the information submitted to FDA;
  - Does not raise new questions of safety and effectiveness; and
  - Demonstrates that the device is at least as safe and effective as the predicate.

Submitters will have to compare their device with similar predicate devices and support their claims, however, they need not be identical. Table 4.1 [89] shows the elements that may be taken into consideration for substantial equivalence. The submitter may not market a device until a letter from the FDA declaring that the device is SE is received. The device may be marketed immediately after the 510(k) clearance is obtained. After the 510(k) clearance, the facility in which the medical device is manufactured may be inspected at anytime. If the FDA determines that a device is not SE, the applicant may choose to resubmit another 510(k) with new data, request a Class I or II designation through the *de novo* process, file a reclassification petition, or submit a PMA [25].

510(k) contents and documents

There is no fixed template for a 510(k) submission, thus, Table 4.2 [89] provides the general elements required in a Traditional 510(k) submission as extracted from the FDA Web site [90]. The FDA "recommends" many of the items in the submission that are not reflected individually here because the more complete the 510(k) is, the more likely it will be approved. Other information for 510(k) submission requirements could be found in the 21 CFR 807 Subpart E [91].

General requirements for 510(k) submission (with reference to Table 4.2)
(1) Medical Device User Fee Cover Sheet [MDUFA 510(k) Cover Sheet] Each 510(k) submission must be accompanied with a MDUFA Cover Sheet, which can be

Table 4.1 Elements for SE comparison [89]

Intended use	Indications for use	Target population
Anatomical site	Location of usage	Energy used and/or delivered
Human factors	Design	Performance
Standards	Materials	Effectiveness
Sterility	Chemical composition	Manufacturing process
Labeling	Biocompatibility	
Safety • Chemical • Electrical • Mechanical • Thermal • Radiation	Compatibility with environment and other device(s)	

Table 4.2 General requirements for premarket notification/510(k) submission [89]

1	MDUFA Cover Sheet	Cover Sheet generated at FDA User Fee Web site
2	CDRH Premarket Review Submission Cover Sheet	Appendix I—FDA Form 3514 Optional, if information here is covered in Cover Letter (3)
3	Cover Letter	See Table 4.3
4	Table of Contents	Number pages by sections (1.1,1.2 or 1-1,1-2) Include list of attachments and appendices
5	510(k) Acceptance Checklist	Appendix II—Acceptance Checklist for Traditional 510(k)
6	Indications for Use Statement	FDA Form 3881
7	510(k) Summary or 510(k) Statement	21 CFR 807.92 21 CFR 807.93
8	Truthful and Accurate Statement	21 CFR 807.87(k)—Template provided by FDA
9	Class III Certification and Summary[a]	Only for Class III devices that are not called for PMA. 21 CFR 807.87(j) and 807.94—Template provided by FDA
10	Financial Certification/ Disclosure Statement[a]	Only if clinical studies information is submitted in 510(k)
11	Conformity Declaration and Summary Reports[a]	Only for declaration of conformity to recognized stands, etc. [Mostly for Abbreviated 510(k)]
12	Executive Summary	Brief description that provides overall understanding of device, indications for use, comparison table (device vs. predicate), summary of performance testing
13	Device Description	Narrative and physical description
14	Substantial Equivalence Comparison	See Tables 4.1, 4.4, and 4.11
15	Proposed Labeling	In line with 21 CFR 807.87(e)
16	Sterilization/Shelf Life[a]	Only for devices sold as sterile
17	Biocompatibility[a]	Only for medical devices that come into direct or indirect contact with patients
18	Software[a]	Only for medical devices that require software
19	Electromagnetic Compatibility[a]	Only for medical devices that include electronic component(s)
20	Performance Testing (Bench, Animal, Clinical)[a]	Only if applicable

[a] If applicable to device.

found at the FDA User Fee Web site [92] that will only be available after a disclaimer and login. All outstanding establishment registration fees have to be paid in order to proceed, otherwise, the FDA will not accept the submission. There would be a series of questions and options to answer before a draft of the MDUFA Cover Sheet would be generated.

Table 4.3 **Summary of elements for cover letter [89]**

Elements	Remarks
Submission Date	Month/Day/Year
Label "510(k) Submission"	Traditional, Special, or Abbreviated
Submitter Contact	Name, Address, Phone Number, Fax Number, Email Specify who is the owner of the 510(k) if consultant or third party involved in preparation Clearly identify contact person
Establishment Registration Number	Optional. Required to register prior to importing device or within 30 days of device marketing. Sufficient to state registration intent following FDA clearance
Device Identity	Common and trade (proprietary) name of device, including model number(s)
Classification	Classification name, class of device, product code, and classification panel (if known) If device has not been classified, include statement for that
Purpose/Reason for this 510(k)	New device? Modification of existing device? Previously submitted 510(k) not found SE? (Include previous 510(k) numbers)
Predicate Device Identity	Provide predicate device 510(k) number, trade name, and product code to which SE is claimed
Facility Details	If applicable, provide registration number, name and address of facility used in manufacture of device
Compliance with any special controls	

During submission of the MDUFA Cover Sheet and payment of fees to the FDA, a Payment Identification Number (PIN) would be obtained and that would be used to track the payment. The FY15 User Fees are shown in Table 4.14 [93]. For more detailed step-by-step instructions, please refer to the FDA User Fee Web site [92, 94]. If a 510(k) application is reviewed by an accredited third party, this may be omitted because the third party may charge review fees. Accredited Persons [95], also known as accredited third parties, are people that are authorized by the FDA to conduct the primary review of 510(k)s for eligible devices [96]. This Accredited Persons Program was created by the FDA Modernization Act of 1997 (FDAMA), based on an FDA pilot [97]. For more information, please refer to the FDA guideline "Implementation of Third Party Programs under the FDA Modernization Act of 1997; Final Guidance for Staff, Industry and Third Parties" [98].

(2) CDRH Premarket Review Submission Cover Sheet—FDA Form 3514 This cover sheet is optional if the element of it is covered in the cover letter in the next section. The FDA Form 3514 can be found at the following link: http://www.fda.gov/downloads/AboutFDA/ReportsManualsForms/Forms/UCM080872.pdf

(3) Cover Letter The cover letter [89] should include the following to provide more informative details of the device, company, etc.

(1) State submission as "510(k) Submission" clearly to aid effective distribution of documents to respective offices, with submission date in the following format (month/day/year) and whether the submission is a Traditional, Special, or Abbreviated 510(k).
(2) State submitter's contact details and clearly identify contact person so that the FDA knows who to contact for additional information. Specify owner of the 510(k) if consultant or a third party is involved in preparation of the 510(k).
(3) Establishment registration number is optional for the submission of the 510(k), however, the company would have to register within 30 days of marketing the device or before importing the device. The annual establishment registration fee for Fiscal Year 2015 is $3646.
(4) State the device's common and trade (proprietary) name, including the model number(s). Trade name is the name under which the device would be marketed.
(5) State device classification name, class, classification panel (Figure 4.3) and the three-letter product code, if known. If the device has not been classified by the FDA, include a statement to this effect. An example of a statement could be, "To my knowledge, the FDA has not classified this device. The product code of xxx has been assigned to this device in the Classification Database." Accessories or software of device(s) usually take on the same classification or highest classification of the "parent" device.
(6) State the purpose or reason for the 510(k): New device, modified device, or previously submitted device which has been found to be not SE to the predicate device(s). For any reason, a detailed description should be given along with any other known details, such as previous or related 510(k) number(s).
(7) State the identity of a predicate device(s) that is found to be similar to the device in question, providing its 510(k) number(s), trade name, product code, and any supporting evidence and details.
(8) Facility details (registration number, name, and address) of each facility should be provided if applicable.
(9) Compliance with special controls

(4) Table of Contents A table of contents is recommended for easy reference and to aid an orderly submission, with a list of attachments and appendices. The FDA recommends that pages should be numbered in sections, example, 1.1, 1.2 or 1-1, 1-2.

(5) 510(k) Acceptance Checklist [99] The acceptance checklist is recommended and the template is made available by the FDA; each type of 510(k) has its own respective checklist.

Links:

Acceptance Checklist for Traditional 510(k) http://www.fda.gov/downloads/MedicalDevices/DeviceRegulationandGuidance/GuidanceDocuments/UCM315014.pdf#page=17

Acceptance Checklist for Abbreviated 510(k) http://www.fda.gov/downloads/MedicalDevices/DeviceRegulationandGuidance/GuidanceDocuments/UCM315014.pdf#page=43

Acceptance Checklist for Special 510(k) http://www.fda.gov/downloads/MedicalDevices/DeviceRegulationandGuidance/GuidanceDocuments/UCM315014.pdf#page=70

(6) Statement of Indications for Use The FDA provides a template for this statement (as shown in Figure 4.7 [100]), in which specific indications, clinical settings, target population, anatomical sites, etc. should be described and should be consistent with labeling, advertising, and usage instructions.

DEPARTMENT OF HEALTH AND HUMAN SERVICES Food and Drug Administration **Indications for Use**	Form Approved: OMB No. 0910-0120 Expiration Date: January 31, 2017 *See PRA Statement below.*

510(k) Number *(if known)*

Device Name

Indications for Use *(Describe)*

Type of Use *(Select one or both, as applicable)*

☐ Prescription Use (Part 21 CFR 801 Subpart D) ☐ Over-The-Counter Use (21 CFR 801 Subpart C)

CONTINUE ON A SEPARATE PAGE IF NEEDED.

This section applies only to requirements of the Paperwork Reduction Act of 1995.

DO NOT SEND YOUR COMPLETED FORM TO THE PRA STAFF EMAIL ADDRESS BELOW.

The burden time for this collection of information is estimated to average 79 hours per response, including the time to review instructions, search existing data sources, gather and maintain the data needed and complete and review the collection of information. Send comments regarding this burden estimate or any other aspect of this information collection, including suggestions for reducing this burden, to:

Department of Health and Human Services
Food and Drug Administration
Office of Chief Information Officer
Paperwork Reduction Act (PRA) Staff
PRAStaff@fda.hhs.gov

"An agency may not conduct or sponsor, and a person is not required to respond to, a collection of information unless it displays a currently valid OMB number."

FORM FDA 3881 (8/14) Page 1 of 1 PSC Publishing Services (301) 443-6740 EF

Figure 4.7 FDA Form 3881 – Indications for Use Statement [100].

510(k) Summary Sample

21 CFR 807.92 Content and format of a 510(k) Summary

510(k) Summary

I. SUBMITTER

Device Submitter, Inc.
123 Main Street
Anywhere, MD 01234

Phone: 555-555-1234
Fax: 555-555-0123

Contact Person: John Contact
Date Prepared: January, 16, 2013

(a1) Submitter's details and date of summary prepared

II. DEVICE

Name of Device: Brand X Endoscopic Stapling System, Model x123, Model y456
Common or Usual Name: Endoscopic Stapling System
Classification Name: Endoscope and Accessories (21 CFR 876.1500)
Regulatory Class: II
Product Code: ODE

(a2) Device details

III. PREDICATE DEVICE

Brand Z Endoscopic Plication System, KXXXXXX
The predicated has not been subject to a design-related recall.

No reference devices were used in this submission.

(a3) Predicate device details

IV. DEVICE DESCRIPTION

The Brand X Endoscopic Stapling System consists of a flexible endoscope, an endoscopy suite, and a number of associated accessories. The endoscope and staples are provided sterile (EtO).

Brand X uses an implant (surgical staple) that is delivered by a flexible endoscopy by a surgeon or gastroenterologist for approximating adjoining portions of the esophageal and gastric tissues at the gastroesophageal junction, thereby creating a permanent surgical fundoplication. The system includes an ultrasonic transducer that operates as a range finder for measuring the relative alignment and the distance between the transducer at the tip of the endoscope (the anvil) and the ultrasonic mirror in the cartridge (that includes the staples). The device deploys sets of implantable staples for performing the fundoplication procedure.

The system combines a video camera, an ultrasonic range finder and a surgical stapler in a single unit. The flexible endoscope includes light guides, irrigation, air insufflation and suction channels that terminate the endoscope tip. The stapler portion includes a cartridge that contains sterile 4.8mm standard "B" shaped titanium surgical staples. Model x123 includes five (5) staples per cartridge, while Model y456 contains only four (4). The tip of the endoscope contains an anvil for the staples, as wells as two small stainless steel screws that are extracted from the tip of the endoscope and engage into nuts positioned in the cartridge. The ultrasonic range finder measures the distance between an ultrasonic mirror in the cartridge and the tip of the endoscope. It also verifies alignment between the cartridge and the anvil, before the insertion of the screws.

The endoscopy suite includes the ISL (Insufflation, Suction and Light) console, the CCU (Camera Control Unit) console and a monitor. The ISL console provides suction, insufflation and a white light (Xenon) source for illumination. The CCU console contains a controller for the camera, ultrasonic range finder and sensors that indicate status of the bending angle, screws and fire. The monitor displays patient information, the video image, and the processed data from the controllers such as ultrasonic data, fire status, degree of bending and crew position. A keyboard for entering data during the procedure is also included. The System includes three software applications: the video controller software, the ultrasound controller software, and the ISL controller software. The software systems work in conjunction with the hardware consoles listed above in order to visualize the procedure and deliver the staples. The endoscope is designed for single-patient use, and it is connect to the CCU and ISL consoles via a multi-connector. The endoscope handle contains the controls used by the operator to manipulate the endoscope.

The associated accessories include:

- Irrigation bottle with liquids for irrigation of the camera lens
- Suction canister for extracting liquids during the procedure
- Silicon tubes for connecting the ISL and other accessories to the endoscop
- Disposable air filter of the suction ISL input channel
- Overtube for protecting patient's pharynx

(a4) Description of device, functions, concepts and other properties

V. INDICATIONS FOR USE

The Brand X Stapling System is indicated for the endoscopic placement of surgical staples in the soft tissue of the esophagus and stomach in order to create anterior partial fundoplication for treatment of symptomatic chronic Gastro Esophageal Reflux Disease (GERD) in patients who require and respond to pharmalogical therapy.

The Indications for Use statement for the Brand X device is not identical to the predicate device; however, the differences do not alter the intended therapeutic use of the device nor do they affect the safety and effectiveness of the device relative to the predicate. Both the subject and predicate devices have the same intended used for the treatment of GERD, by approximating tissue in the esophagus and stomach.

(a5) Statement of intended use of the device and description of treatment, etc

VI. COMPARISON OF TECHNOLOGICAL CHARACTERISTICS WITH THE PREDICATE DEVICE

Transoral endoscopic fundoplication is the technological principle for both the subject and predicate devices. It is based on the use of endoscopic instrumentation for approximating and permanently adjoining gastric and esophageal tissues, creating plications at the level of the gastroesophageal valve and thereby restoring valvular functionality and reducing gastric reflux into the esophagus.
At a high level, the subject and predicate devices are based on the following same technological elements:
Endoscope – used to reach the target tissue
Device inserted through an overtube – to protect the esophagus
Creation of a gastric (or gastroesophageal) plication in close proximity to the gastroesophageal junction by the retroflexed device
Use of a permanent implant to secure tissue
Use of a mechanical component for positioning and launching the implant
User-controlled mechanical trigger (or knob) to launch the fastener (implant)
Mechanically securing the plication by a permanent implant fastener

The following technological differences exist between the subject and predicate devices:
Use of an ultrasound range finder
Use of a staple as a fastener
Use of a different tissue capture and fixation mechanisms
The predicate device must be used in conjunction with a flexible endoscope whereas the subject device has a flexible endoscope incorporated into the system.

(a6) Comparison of technological characteristics (i.e., design, material, chemical composition, energy source)

(Continued)

(7) 510(k) Summary or Statement Content and format of the 510(k) summary is according to 21 CFR 807 Subpart E Section 807.92 [101].

A sample of the 510(k) Summary provided by the FDA guidance documents [102] is as follows:

Content and format of 510(k) statement is according to 21 CFR 807 Subpart E Section 807.93 [103].

The 510(k) Statement template [104] provided by the FDA is as follows:

——————— Template for 510(k) Statement (Start) ———————

510(k) Statement

(As Required By 21 CFR 807.93)

I certify that, in my capacity as (*the position held in company by person required to submit the premarket notification, preferably the official correspondent*) of (*company name*), I will make available all information included in this premarket notification on safety and effectiveness within 30 days of request by any person if the device described in the premarket notification submission is determined to be substantially equivalent. The information I agree to make available will be a duplicate of the premarket notification submission, including any adverse safety and effectiveness information, but excluding all patient identifiers, and trade secret and confidential commercial information, as defined in 21 CFR 20.61.

VII. PERFORMANCE DATA

The following performance data were provided in support of the substantial equivalence determination.

Biocompatibility testing

The biocompatibility evaluation for the Brand X device was conducted in accordance with the FDA Blue Book Memorandum #G95-1 "Use of International Standard ISO-10993, 'Biological Evaluation of Medical Devices Part 1: Evaluation and Testing,'" May 1, 1995, and International Standard ISO 10993-1 "Biological Evaluation of Medical Devices – Part 1: Evaluation and Testing Within a Risk Management Process," as recognized by FDA. The battery of testing included the following tests:

- Cytotoxicity
- Sensitization
- Irritation
- Systemic toxicity
- Pyrogen Testing

The endoscopic delivery system is considered tissue contacting for a duration of less than 24 hours, while the staples are considered permanent implants. The titanium staple material conforms to ASTM F-67-06 for chemical composition.

Electrical safety and electromagnetic compatibility (EMC)

Electrical safety and EMC testing were conducted on the Brand X device, consisting of the ISL console, CCU console and endoscope. The system complies with the IEC 60601-1, IEC 60601-2-18 and IEC 60601-2-37 standards for safety and the IEC 60601-1-2 standard for EMC.

Software verification and validation testing

Software verification and validation testing were conducted and documentation was provided as recommended by FDA's Guidance for Industry and FDA Staff, "Guidance for the Content of Premarket Submissions for Software Contained in Medical Devices." The software for this device was considered as a "major" level of concern, since a failure or latent flaw in the software could directly result in serious injury or death to the patient or operator.

Mechanical and acoustic testing

- Acoustic testing
- Elongation of the bending cable
- Torque on the handle wheel and force on cable
- Crimp assembly, cable tensile strength, cable flexibility, minimum bending radius of the cables
- Staple verification
- Simulated use testing

Animal study

In the animal study conducted, 16 pigs underwent endoscopy with the Brand X System. 12 pigs underwent fundoplication, and 4 pigs served as a sham (control) group. There were no procedure related complications or premature deaths in this study, at the 2, 4 and 6 week follow-up (4 pigs in each group).

The safety and feasibility of the Brand X device were evaluated by macroscopic and histological evaluation of the tissue in the treatment stapled areas. These studies demonstrated that the Brand X device can safely create and anterior partial fundoplication, similar to that which is constructed using other endoscopic suturing devices.

(b1) Discussion of nonclinical tests submitted or referenced

(Continued)

Clinical studies
Clinical testing of the Brand X device included an initial feasibility study of 6 patients, a pilot study consisting of 13 patients and a pivotal study of 72 patients. Substantial equivalence was based in part on the pivotal study.

Pivotal Study
The pivotal study was a prospective, multi-center, open label, non-randomized, single arm study of 72 patients, of which 66 were available for primary endpoint analysis; 3 subjects did not complete the procedure, and 3 were excluded from the effectiveness analysis. The device was used to staple the fundus of the stomach to the esophagus, using standard B shaped surgical staples. Stapling was performed in two or three locations at least 1.5 cm above the GE junction, separated by at least 90 degrees. The procedure was intended to create a partial anterior fundoplication as a reflux barrier. Patients were followed for a period of six months at 6 sites both in the United States and outside of the United States under IDE G070136.

Primary effectiveness endpoint:
GERD health related quality of life score (GERD-HRQL) off proton pump inhibitor (PPI) was improved from baseline by >50%, at six months post procedure in at least 53% of the patients (53% is the lower boundary of the 95% confidence interval).

Primary safety endpoint:
The primary safety endpoint consisted of all treatment-related adverse events, during and after the procedure. "Treatment-related" events were conventionally defined as those which occurred in the first 30 days post-procedure.

Effectiveness
The primary endpoint for the Brand X study focused on the GERD-HRQL score. The study results demonstrated that 75% of the patients had a >50% improvement in their GERD-HRQL score off PPI at six months compared to baseline. Hence the study met its primary endpoint with the required 95% confidence level.

(b2) Discussion of clinical tests submitted or referenced

The reduction in the median score for the Brand X device of 23.0 units (from 29.0 to 6.0) represents a
79.3% improvement. This value is almost identical to the published result for the pivotal trial of the predicate device (79.2%). Therefore, the effectiveness of the Brand X system in successfully treating chronic symptoms of GERD is similar to the effectiveness reported for the predicate device.

(b2) Discussion of clinical tests submitted or referenced

The median value of the percent of time pH < 4.0 decreased from an initial value of 8.3% at baseline to 6.75%. Therefore, the study met its secondary endpoint related to the acid exposure test. A comparison to results reported in the literature revealed that the change in the median values of the Brand X device showed a decrease of 19%, while the predicate showed a decrease of 18%. Hence, the Brand X results in reducing the exposure to gastric acids are similar to those reported for the predicate system.

Safety
The study reported nine patients with a total of nine serious adverse events (SAEs). Four events were considered mild in intensity, involving pain and fever. Three events were classified as moderate in intensity, involving pneumothorax, pneumomediastinum, and pneumoperitoneum (all resolved spontaneously). Two events were considered severe in intensity: one involved esophageal perforation (required drainage) and another had suicidal thoughts (non-device/procedure related).

Six of the SAEs were considered related to the device: one definitely (esophageal perforation) and the others possibly. Three events were considered not related to the device. The median time from procedure to SAE was 1.5 days for events related to the device. None of the patients with SAEs required any operation or re-operation. Adverse events reported that occurred in greater than the 5% level were postoperative pain or discomfort in 33% of patients, postoperative nausea in approximately 10%, and sore throat in 21%. The adverse events were mild or insignificant in most cases.

The SAEs and overall safety profile were similar to the predicate device for which two perforations and one bleeding event were reported. The number of AEs was similar to those reported for the predicate device. Three cases of fever were reported in the current study (for 72 patients), similar to the 3 cases of fever reported for the predicate. There were 23 cases of chest pain (23/72 = 32%) vs.
17% reported for the predicate; abdominal pain was recorded for 5% of the patients in the current study vs. 44% of the patients for the predicate. Sore throat was reported for 15 patients (15/72 = 21%) vs. 15% for the predicate.

(b2) Discussion of clinical tests submitted or referenced (cont'd)

<u>Summary</u>
Based on the clinical performance as documented in the pivotal clinical study, the Brand X system was found to have a safety and effectiveness profile that is similar to the predicate device.

VIII. CONCLUSIONS

Since the predicate device was cleared based in part on the results of clinical studies, and since the comparison of bench testing to clinical outcomes is still not well understood for this type of device, clinical testing was required to support substantial equivalence. The non-clinical data support the safety of the device and the hardware and software verification and validation demonstrate that the Brand X device should perform as intended in the specified use conditions. The clinical data demonstrate that the Brand X device performs comparably to the predicate device that is currently marketed for the same intended use.

(b3) Conclusions drawn from tests

____

(Signature of Certifier)

____

(Typed Name)

____

(Date)

____

*(Premarket Notification [510(k)] Number)
*For a new submission, leave the 510(k) number blank.

——— Template for 510(k) Statement (End) ———

(8) Truthful and Accurate Statement This statement is to certify that all information submitted is truthful and accurate, and it may be included in the 510(k) cover letter or separately on its own. If the CDRH Premarket Review Submission Cover Sheet is used, this statement should be attached as a separate sheet.

The Truthful and Accurate Statement template [105] provided by the FDA is as follows:

———————————————— Template for Truthful and Accurate Statement (Start) ————————————————

Truthful and Accurate Statement

[As Required by 21 CFR 807.87(k)]

I certify that, in my capacity as (*the position held in company*) of (*company name*), I believe to the best of my knowledge, that all data and information submitted in the premarket notification are truthful and accurate and that no material fact has been omitted.

____

(Signature)

____

(Typed Name)

____

(Date)

____

*(Premarket Notification [510(k)] Number)

*For a new submission, leave the 510(k) number blank. Must be signed by a responsible person of the firm required to submit the premarket notification [e.g., not a consultant for the 510(k) submitter].

———————— Template for Truthful and Accurate Statement (Start) ————————

(9) Class III Certification and Summary (if applicable) In accordance with 21 CFR 807.87(j) and 807.94, submitter is required to certify the following only if claiming substantial equivalence to a device which has been classified as Class III.

The Class III Certification and Summary template [106] provided by the FDA is as follows:

———————— Template for Premarket Notification Class III Certification and Summary (Start) ————————

Premarket Notification Class III Certification and Summary

(As Required by 21 CFR 807.94)

(To be submitted when claiming equivalence to a Class III device)

I certify that, in my capacity as (*the position held in company*) of (*company name*) that I have conducted a reasonable search of all information known or otherwise available about the types and causes of safety and/or effectiveness problems that have been reported for the (*device name*). I further certifiy that I am aware of the types of problems to which the (*device name*) is susceptible and that, to the best of my knowledge, the following summary of the types and causes of safety and/or effectiveness problems about the (*device name*) is complete and accurate.

(Attach the summary of problem data, bibliography or other citations upon which the summary is based.)

____

(Signature of Certifier)

____

(Typed Name)

____

(Date)

____

*(Premarket Notification [510(k)] Number)

*For a new submission, leave the 510(k) number blank. Must be signed by a responsible person of the firm required to submit the premarket notification [e.g., not a consultant for the 510(k) submitter].

——————— Template for Premarket Notification Class III Certification and Summary (End) ———————

(10) Financial Certification or Disclosure Statement (if applicable) As stated in 21 CFR 807.87(i), a financial certification and/or disclosure statement for each clinical investigator must be submitted only if information from clinical studies for the 510(k) is to be submitted [90]. FDA Form 3454 and Form 3455 are shown in Figures 4.8 and 4.9, respectively.

(11) Conformity Declaration and Summary Reports (if applicable) The conformity declaration and summary reports are usually required when submitting an Abbreviated 510(k), where there are declarations of conformity to recognized standards or guidance. A Standards Data Report form (Figure 4.10a and b) is provided by the FDA for referring to a national or international standard.

Related guidance

- Guidance for Industry and FDA Staff—Recognition and Use of Consensus Standards [107]
- Guidance for Industry and FDA Staff—Use of Standards in Substantial Equivalence Determinations [108]

(12) Executive Summary An Executive Summary should include a brief description of the overall understanding of the device, indications for use and technology, Substantial Equivalence (SE) comparison with predicate, brief summary of performance testing with methods used, and any conclusions drawn.

(13) Device Description Performance specifications and a brief description of device design is required, with models and accessories and/or components, if applicable. Drawings of the device with measurements and/or schematics, and other supporting details would aid in the full description of the device.

(14) Substantial Equivalence (SE) Comparison Before comparison, the predicate device would have to be identified with its trade name, model number, 510(k) number, etc., if available. More than one predicate device may be used.

Table 4.1 shows the usual elements considered for SE comparison for a device and its predicate. The FDA helps to simplify the SE decision-making process with Table 4.4 [109] and Figure 4.11. Table 4.4 and Figure 4.11 are essentially asking the same questions as noted by steps in the table and points in the flowchart. SE/NSE determination of a medical device may be concluded by following through with the steps or points.

DEPARTMENT OF HEALTH AND HUMAN SERVICES
Food and Drug Administration

CERTIFICATION: FINANCIAL INTERESTS AND ARRANGEMENTS OF CLINICAL INVESTIGATORS

Form Approved: OMB No. 0910-0396
Expiration Date: December 31, 2015

TO BE COMPLETED BY APPLICANT

With respect to all covered clinical studies (or specific clinical studies listed below (if appropriate)) submitted in support of this application, I certify to one of the statements below as appropriate. I understand that this certification is made in compliance with 21 CFR part 54 and that for the purposes of this statement, a clinical investigator includes the spouse and each dependent child of the investigator as defined in 21 CFR 54.2(d).

Please mark the applicable check box.

☐ (1) As the sponsor of the submitted studies, I certify that I have not entered into any financial arrangement with the listed clinical investigators (enter names of clinical investigators below or attach list of names to this form) whereby the value of compensation to the investigator could be affected by the outcome of the study as defined in 21 CFR 54.2(a). I also certify that each listed clinical investigator required to disclose to the sponsor whether the investigator had a proprietary interest in this product or a significant equity in the sponsor as defined in 21 CFR 54.2(b) did not disclose any such interests. I further certify that no listed investigator was the recipient of significant payments of other sorts as defined in 21 CFR 54.2(f).

Clinical Investigators		

☐ (2) As the applicant who is submitting a study or studies sponsored by a firm or party other than the applicant, I certify that based on information obtained from the sponsor or from participating clinical investigators, the listed clinical investigators (attach list of names to this form) did not participate in any financial arrangement with the sponsor of a covered study whereby the value of compensation to the investigator for conducting the study could be affected by the outcome of the study (as defined in 21 CFR 54.2(a)); had no proprietary interest in this product or significant equity interest in the sponsor of the covered study (as defined in 21 CFR 54.2(b)); and was not the recipient of significant payments of other sorts (as defined in 21 CFR 54.2(f)).

☐ (3) As the applicant who is submitting a study or studies sponsored by a firm or party other than the applicant, I certify that I have acted with due diligence to obtain from the listed clinical investigators (attach list of names) or from the sponsor the information required under 54.4 and it was not possible to do so. The reason why this information could not be obtained is attached.

NAME	TITLE
FIRM/ORGANIZATION	
SIGNATURE	DATE *(mm/dd/yyyy)*

This section applies only to the requirements of the Paperwork Reduction Act of 1995.
An agency may not conduct or sponsor, and a person is not required to respond to, a collection of information unless it displays a currently valid OMB control number. Public reporting burden for this collection of information is estimated to average 1 hour per response, including time for reviewing instructions, searching existing data sources, gathering and maintaining the necessary data, and completing and reviewing the collection of information. Send comments regarding this burden estimate or any other aspect of this collection of information to the address to the right:

Do NOT send your completed form to the PRA Staff email address below.
Department of Health and Human Services
Food and Drug Administration
Office of Chief Information Officer
PRAStaff@fda.hhs.gov

"An agency may not conduct or sponsor, and a person is not required to respond to, a collection of information unless it displays a currently valid OMB number."

FORM FDA 3454 (4/13) PSC Publishing Services (301) 443-6740 EF

Figure 4.8 FDA Form 3454—Certification: Financial Interests and Arrangements of Clinical Investigators.

DEPARTMENT OF HEALTH AND HUMAN SERVICES
Food and Drug Administration

DISCLOSURE: FINANCIAL INTERESTS AND ARRANGEMENTS OF CLINICAL INVESTIGATORS

Form Approved: OMB No. 0910-0396
Expiration Date: December 31, 2015

TO BE COMPLETED BY APPLICANT

The following information concerning ______________________ (*Name of clinical investigator*), who participated as a clinical investigator in the submitted study ______________________ (*Name of clinical study*) is submitted in accordance with 21 CFR part 54. The named individual has participated in financial arrangements or holds financial interests that are required to be disclosed as follows:

Please mark the applicable check boxes.

- ☐ any financial arrangement entered into between the sponsor of the covered study and the clinical investigator involved in the conduct of the covered study, whereby the value of the compensation to the clinical investigator for conducting the study could be influenced by the outcome of the study;
- ☐ any significant payments of other sorts made on or after February 2, 1999, from the sponsor of the covered study, such as a grant to fund ongoing research, compensation in the form of equipment, retainer for ongoing consultation, or honoraria;
- ☐ any proprietary interest in the product tested in the covered study held by the clinical investigator;
- ☐ any significant equity interest, as defined in 21 CFR 54.2(b), held by the clinical investigator in the sponsor of the covered study.

Details of the individual's disclosable financial arrangements and interests are attached, along with a description of steps taken to minimize the potential bias of clinical study results by any of the disclosed arrangements or interests.

NAME	TITLE
FIRM/ORGANIZATION	
SIGNATURE	Date *(mm/dd/yyyy)*

This section applies only to the requirements of the Paperwork Reduction Act of 1995.

An agency may not conduct or sponsor, and a person is not required to respond to, a collection of information unless it displays a currently valid OMB control number. Public reporting burden for this collection of information is estimated to average 5 hours per response, including time for reviewing instructions, searching existing data sources, gathering and maintaining the necessary data, and completing and reviewing the collection of information. Send comments regarding this burden estimate or any other aspect of this collection of information to the address to the right:

Do NOT send your completed form to the PRA Staff email address below.

Department of Health and Human Services
Food and Drug Administration
Office of Chief Information Officer
PRAStaff@fda.hhs.gov

"An agency may not conduct or sponsor, and a person is not required to respond to, a collection of information unless it displays a currently valid OMB number."

FORM FDA 3455 (4/13) PSC Publishing Services (301) 443-6740 EF

Figure 4.9 FDA Form 3455—Disclosure: Financial Interests and Arrangements of Clinical Investigators.

Form Approved: OMB No. 0910-0120; Expiration Date: 1/31/2017

Department of Health and Human Services
Food and Drug Administration

STANDARDS DATA REPORT FOR 510(k)s

(To be filled in by applicant)

This report and the Summary Report Table are to be completed by the applicant when submitting a 510(k) that references a national or international standard. A separate report is required for each standard referenced in the 510(k).

TYPE OF 510(K) SUBMISSION

☐ Traditional ☐ Special ☐ Abbreviated

STANDARD TITLE [1]

Please answer the following questions	Yes	No
Is this standard recognized by FDA [2]?	☐	☐
FDA Recognition number [3]	#______	
Was a third party laboratory responsible for testing conformity of the device to this standard identified in the 510(k)?	☐	☐
Is a summary report [4] describing the extent of conformance of the standard used included in the 510(k)? If no, complete a summary report table.	☐	☐
Does the test data for this device demonstrate conformity to the requirements of this standard as it pertains to this device?	☐	☐
Does this standard include acceptance criteria? If no, include the results of testing in the 510(k).	☐	☐
Does this standard include more than one option or selection of tests? If yes, report options selected in the summary report table.	☐	☐
Were there any deviations or adaptations made in the use of the standard?	☐	☐
If yes, were deviations in accordance with the FDA supplemental information sheet (SIS) [5]?	☐	☐
Were deviations or adaptations made beyond what is specified in the FDA SIS? If yes, report these deviations or adaptations in the summary report table.	☐	☐
Were there any exclusions from the standard? If yes, report these exclusions in the summary report table.	☐	☐
Is there an FDA guidance [6] that is associated with this standard?	☐	☐
If yes, was the guidance document followed in preparation of this 510k?	☐	☐
Title of guidance: ______		

[1] The formatting convention for the title is: [SDO] [numeric identifier] [title of standard] [date of publication]

[2] Authority [21 U.S.C. 360d], http://www.fda.gov/MedicalDevices/DeviceRegulationandGuidance/Standards/default.htm

[3] http://www.accessdata.fda.gov/scripts/cdrh/cfdocs/cfStandards/search.cfm

[4] The summary report should include: any adaptations used to adapt to the device under review (for example, alternative test methods); choices made when options or a selection of methods are described; deviations from the standard; requirements not applicable to the device; and the name and address of the test laboratory or certification body involved in conformance assessment to this standard. The summary report includes information on all standards utilized during the development of the device.

[5] The supplemental information sheet (SIS) is additional information which is necessary before FDA recognizes the standard. Found at http://www.accessdata.fda.gov/scripts/cdrh/cfdocs/cfStandards/search.cfm

[6] The online search for CDRH Guidance Documents can be found at http://www.fda.gov/MedicalDevices/DeviceRegulationandGuidance/GuidanceDocuments/default.htm

FORM FDA 3654 (4/14) Page 1 of 2 PSC Publishing Services (301) 443-6740 EF

Figure 4.10 (a) FDA Form 3654—Standards Data Report for 510(k)s (Page 1/2) and

EXTENT OF STANDARD CONFORMANCE SUMMARY REPORT TABLE		
STANDARD TITLE		
CONFORMANCE WITH STANDARD SECTIONS*		
SECTION NUMBER	SECTION TITLE	CONFORMANCE? ☐ Yes ☐ No ☐ N/A
TYPE OF DEVIATION OR OPTION SELECTED ◆		
DESCRIPTION		
JUSTIFICATION		
SECTION NUMBER	SECTION TITLE	CONFORMANCE? ☐ Yes ☐ No ☐ N/A
TYPE OF DEVIATION OR OPTION SELECTED ◆		
DESCRIPTION		
JUSTIFICATION		
SECTION NUMBER	SECTION TITLE	CONFORMANCE? ☐ Yes ☐ No ☐ N/A
TYPE OF DEVIATION OR OPTION SELECTED ◆		
DESCRIPTION		
JUSTIFICATION		

* For completeness list all sections of the standard and indicate whether conformance is met. If a section is not applicable (N/A) an explanation is needed under "justification." Some standards include options, so similar to deviations, the option chosen needs to be described and adequately justified as appropriate for the subject device. Explanation of all deviations or description of options selected when following a standard is required under "type of deviation or option selected," "description" and "justification" on the report. More than one page may be necessary.

◆ Types of deviations can include an exclusion of a section in the standard, a deviation brought out by the FDA supplemental information sheet (SIS), a deviation to adapt the standard to the device, or any adaptation of a section.

This section applies only to requirements of the Paperwork Reduction Act of 1995.

DO NOT SEND YOUR COMPLETED FORM TO THE PRA STAFF EMAIL ADDRESS BELOW.

The burden time for this collection of information is estimated to average 1 hour per response, including the time to review instructions, search existing data sources, gather and maintain the data needed and complete and review the collection of information. Send comments regarding this burden estimate or any other aspect of this information collection, including suggestions for reducing this burden, to:

Department of Health and Human Services
Food and Drug Administration
Office of Chief Information Officer
Paperwork Reduction Act (PRA) Staff
PRAStaff@fda.hhs.gov

"An agency may not conduct or sponsor, and a person is not required to respond to, a collection of information unless it displays a currently valid OMB control number."

FORM FDA 3654 (4/14) Page 2 of 2 Add page

Figure 4.10 Continued (b) FDA Form 3654—Standards Data Report for 510(k)s (Page 2/2).

Table 4.4 Substantial equivalence decision-making process [109]

Step	Description	Next step
1	Is product a device?	If YES, go to next step If NO, Stop (not device)
2	Is device subject to 510(k)?	If YES, go to next step If NO, Stop [not 510(k)]
3	Does new device have same indication statement as predicate?	If YES, go to Step 5 If NO, go to next step
4	Do differences in indication statement raise new issues of safety or effectiveness?	If YES, Stop → NSE If NO, go to next step
5	Does new device have same technological characteristics as predicate?	If YES, go to Step 7 If NO, go to next step
6	Could new technological characteristics affect safety or effectiveness?	If YES, go to Step 8 If NO, go to next step
7	Are descriptive characteristics precise enough to ensure equivalence?	If YES, Stop → SE If NO, go to Step 10
8	Are there any new types of safety or effectiveness questions?	If YES, Stop → NSE If NO, go to next step
9	Are there any accepted scientific methods that exist?	If YES, go to next step If NO, Stop → NSE
10	Are performance data available?	If YES, go to next step If NO, Request Data
11	Do data demonstrate equivalence?	If YES, Final Decision → SE If NO, Stop → NSE

NSE: not substantial equivalence; SE: substantial equivalence.

(15) Proposed Labeling Copies of proposed labels, packaging inserts, and all label-related materials must be included in the 510(k). Although the material on which it is printed need not be the actual material used, the labeling has to be the final draft. Copies of labeling for the predicate device(s) are recommended to be submitted as well. Labeling requirements can be found in 21 CFR 801 [110] and Device Labeling Guidance #G91-1 (blue book memo) [111].

(16–20) Additional Requirements (if applicable) Additional requirements items 16–20 are required only if applicable. Table 4.5 provides links to any guidance or forms if available.

Contents for other 510(k)s

The basic requirements for submission of an Abbreviated 510(k) and a Special 510(k) are similar to the Traditional 510(k). As mentioned earlier, the FDA uses the 510(k) paradigm (Figure 4.6) to develop the Abbreviated 510(k) and Special 510(k) to streamline the 510(k) review process, giving submitters some incentive to use a

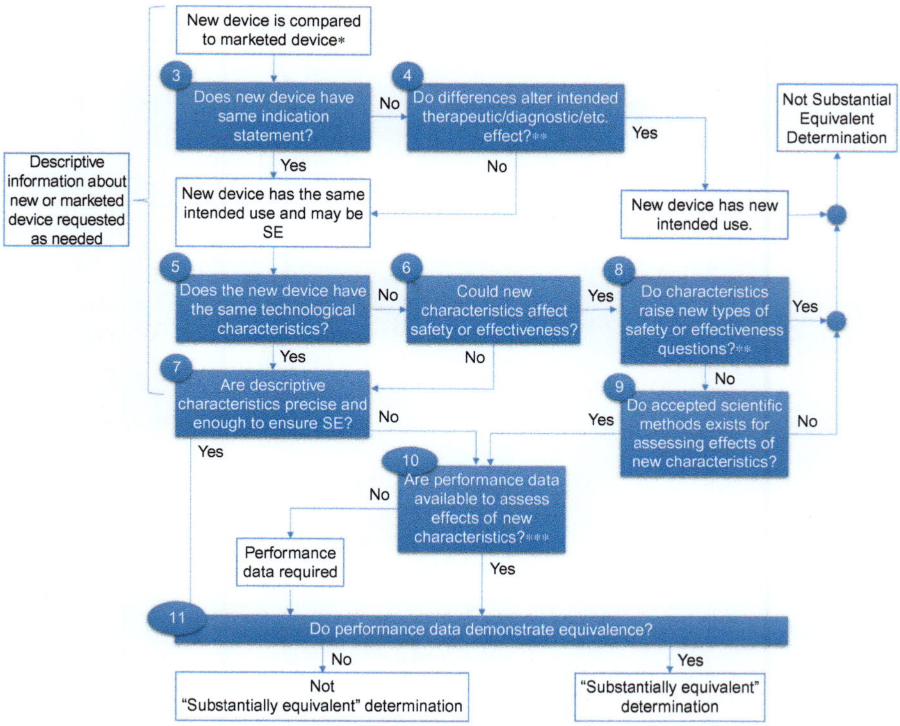

Figure 4.11 510(k) Substantial Equivalence Decision-Making Process Flowchart [90]. *510(k) submissions compare new devices to marketed devices. The FDA requests additional information if the relationship between marketed and "predicate" (preamendments or reclassified postamendments) devices is unclear. **This decision is normally based on descriptive information alone, but limited testing information is sometimes required. ***Data may be in the 510(k), other 510(k)s, the Center's classification files, or the literature.

different submission, instead of the usual Traditional 510(k). For example, the FDA established a 30 day review clock for Special 510(k), shortening the average 3 months for a normal 510(k) clearance. The differences between the three types of 510(k) submissions are depicted in Table 4.6.

The Abbreviated 510(k) relies on the use of special controls and recognized standards and guidance. Thus, the FDA has developed many device-specific guidance documents [112] to aid in the submission of the Abbreviated 510(k). Special controls are used as a means to prove that the safety and effectiveness of a device can be assured by addressing a specific risk or issue. The device must conform to either relevant guidance documents or FDA recognized consensus standards, or both. These consensus standards are either part or all of national and international standards recognized by the FDA. FDA recognized standards usually include specific acceptance benchmarks of relevant performance characteristics of a specific medical device. Thus, conforming to the standards would reduce the amount of data and documentation needed, therefore reducing review time. Currently, the FDA has recognized about 400 standards and a list of current FDA recognized

Table 4.5 **Information for additional requirements**

16	Sterilization/Shelf Life	*Only for devices sold as sterile.* Updated 510(k) Sterility Review Guidance K90-1; Final Guidance for Industry and FDA: http://www.fda.gov/MedicalDevices/DeviceRegulationandGuidance/GuidanceDocuments/ucm072783.htm Guidance for Industry and FDA Staff—Medical Devices User Fee and Modernization Act of 2002, Validation Data in Premarket Notification Submissions [510(k)s] for Reprocessed Single-Use Medical Devices: http://www.fda.gov/MedicalDevices/DeviceRegulationandGuidance/GuidanceDocuments/ucm071434.htm
17	Biocompatibility	*Only for medical devices that come into direct or indirect contact with patients.* Use of International Standard ISO-10993, "Biological Evaluation of Medical Devices Part 1: Evaluation and Testing" (Replaces #G87-1 #8294)(blue book memo): http://www.fda.gov/MedicalDevices/DeviceRegulationandGuidance/GuidanceDocuments/ucm080735.htm
18	Software	*Only for medical devices that require software.* Guidance for the Content of Premarket Submissions for Software Contained in Medical Devices: http://www.fda.gov/MedicalDevices/DeviceRegulationandGuidance/GuidanceDocuments/ucm089543.htm
19	Electromagnetic Compatibility	*Only for medical devices that include electronic component(s).* Electromagnetic Compatibility (EMC): http://www.fda.gov/Radiation-EmittingProducts/RadiationSafety/ElectromagneticCompatibilityEMC/default.htm FDA recommends to use following for device testing: IEC 60601-1-2 Medical Electrical Equipment—Part 1: General Requirements for Safety; Electromagnetic Compatibility—Requirements and Tests (Second Edition, 2001) or equivalent
20	Performance Testing (Bench, Animal, Clinical)	*Only if applicable.* Guidance for performance testing may be found in the Guidance for Industry and FDA Staff: Format for Traditional and Abbreviated 510(k)s: http://www.fda.gov/MedicalDevices/DeviceRegulationandGuidance/GuidanceDocuments/ucm084365.htm

Table 4.5 Continued

	Others	*Convenience Kits* Convenience Kits interim Regulatory Guidance: http://www.fda.gov/MedicalDevices/DeviceRegulationandGuidance/GuidanceDocuments/ucm080216.htm Sterilized Convenience Kits for Clinical and Surgical Use: http://www.fda.gov/MedicalDevices/DeviceRegulationandGuidance/GuidanceDocuments/ucm071019.htm Kit Certification for 510(k)s: http://www.fda.gov/MedicalDevices/DeviceRegulationandGuidance/GuidanceDocuments/ucm080213.htm

standards can be found at the FDA—Recognized Consensus Standards page [113]. In addition, a summary report is required for submission, to demonstrate adherence to the guidance documents, recognized standards, and/or special controls. These allow the FDA to review more efficiently and lead to faster 510(k) clearance.

The Special 510(k) makes use of certain features of QSR and so for the Special 510(k) submission method, manufacturers must first ensure that the risk analysis, necessary verification, and validation activities are conducted to prove that the modified device design output meet the design input requirements. Upon satisfactory completion of this process,

Table 4.6 Which 510(k) to use?

Traditional 510(k)	Abbreviated 510(k)	Special 510(k)
May be used under any circumstances, including other significant modification where Special 510(k) cannot be used.	For device that conforms with: • FDA device specific guidance documents • Special controls • Recognized consensus standards The standards/controls must be used in the 510(k) to be considered an Abbreviated 510(k).	For own marketed device modifications that include: • Energy type • Environmental specifications • Performance specifications • Ergonomics of the patient-user interface • Dimensional specifications • Software or firmware • Packaging or expiration dating • Sterilization

a Special 510(k): Device Modification may then be submitted. Special 510(k)s are usually used when there is a minor modification that does not change the intended use or alter the fundamental scientific technology of an already legally marketed device, hence the cleared 510(k) number must be included in the submission. Some of the modifications are listed in Table 4.6 and they have to adhere closely to the QSR design controls. In addition, the FDA provides a comprehensive guidance for “Deciding When to Submit a 510 (k) for a Change to an Existing Device (K97-1)” [114] to help with decision making.

Table 4.6 summarizes the submission documents for the three types of 510(k)s. Submission documents are mainly similar except for the last few items (Table 4.7).

For declaration of conformity to recognized consensus standards for Abbreviated 510 (k), the following elements in Table 4.8 are required, as provided by the FDA [115]. For the declaration of conformity with design controls for Special 510(k), the declaration should be signed by the designated individual(s) responsible and should include:

Table 4.7 Content for the different types of 510(k)s

Traditional 510(k)	Abbreviated 510(k)	Special 510(k)
MDUFA Cover Sheet		
CDRH Premarket Review Submission Cover Sheet		
Cover Letter		
Table of Contents		
510(k) Acceptance Checklist [for respective 510(k)s]—*see Appendices IIa, IIb and IIc.*		
Indications for Use Statement		
510(k) Summary or 510(k) Statement		
Truthful and Accurate Statement		
Class III Certification and Summary[a]		
Financial Certification/Disclosure Statement[a]		
Executive Summary		
Device Description		
Substantial Equivalence Comparison		
Proposed Labeling		
Sterilization/Shelf Life[a]		
Biocompatibility[a]		
Software[a]		
Electromagnetic Compatibility[a]		
Performance Testing (Bench, Animal, Clinical)[a]		
Not applicable	Conformity Declaration and Summary Reports	Conformity Declaration with design control requirements
	Not Applicable	Certification of Compliance FDA Form 3674
		Standards Data Report[a] FDA Form 3654

[a]Only if applicable to device.

Table 4.8 Required elements for a declaration of conformity to a recognized standard

Required element	Present	Inadequate/ missing
a. An identification of the applicable recognized consensus standards that were met. b. A statement, for each consensus standard, that all requirements were met, except for inapplicable requirements or deviations noted below. c. An identification, for each consensus standard, of any way (s) in which the standard may have been adapted for application to the device under review (e.g., an identification of an alternative series of tests that were performed). d. An identification, for each consensus standard, of any requirements that were not applicable to the device. e. A specification of any deviations from each applicable standard that were applied. f. A specification of the differences that may exist, if any, between the tested device and the device to be marketed and a justification of the test results in these areas of difference. g. The name and address of the testing laboratory and/or certification body involved in determining the conformance of the device with applicable consensus standards and a reference to any accreditations for those organizations.		

a. A statement that, as required by the risk analysis, all verification and validation activities were performed by the designated individual(s) and the results demonstrated that the predetermined acceptance criteria were met; and

b. A statement that the manufacturing facility is in conformance with the design control procedure requirements as specified in 21 CFR 820.30 and the records are available for review.

The templates for the Certification of Compliance (Figure 4.12a and b) and the Standards Data Report (only if national or international standard is used) (Figure 4.10a and b) are provided by the FDA [116].

4.2.3.3 Class III process—PMA

For medical devices which fall under Class III, PMN 510(k) may not be stringent enough for a device with high risk, for example, a defibrillator, or devices that are more critical or used to sustain human life. In this sense, 510(k) based on substantial equivalence is established on descriptive information and emphasis on labeling evaluation, while PMA is dependent on performance data. Table 4.9 shows basic comparison of a 510(k) and a PMA. Unless exempted or otherwise stated in the CFR, device manufacturers for Class III devices (and some Class II devices) would need to apply for PMA approval before being able to market the device.

Form Approved: OMB No. 0910-0616. Expiration Date: 2/28/2015. See PRA Statement on page 2.

FDA

DEPARTMENT OF HEALTH AND HUMAN SERVICES
Food and Drug Administration

Certification of Compliance

Under 42 U.S.C. § 282(j)(5)(B), with Requirements of ClinicalTrials.gov Data Bank (42 U.S.C. § 282(j))

(For submission with an application/submission, including amendments, supplements, and resubmissions, under §§ 505, 515, 520(m), or 510(k) of the Federal Food, Drug, and Cosmetic Act or § 351 of the Public Health Service Act.)

SPONSOR / APPLICANT / SUBMITTER INFORMATION

1. Name of Sponsor/Applicant/Submitter

2. Date of the Application/Submission Which This Certification Accompanies

3. Address
   - Address 1 *(Street address, P.O. box, company name c/o)*
   - Address 2 *(Apartment, suite, unit, building, floor, etc.)*
   - City
   - State/Province/Region
   - Country
   - ZIP or Postal Code

4. Telephone and Fax Numbers *(Include country code if applicable and area code)*
   (Tel): __________
   (Fax): __________

PRODUCT INFORMATION

5. **For Drugs/Biologics:** Include Any/All Available Established, Proprietary and/or Chemical/Biochemical/Blood/Cellular/Gene Therapy Product Name(s).
   For Devices: Include Any/All Common or Usual Name(s), Classification, Trade or Proprietary or Model Name(s) and/or Model Number(s)

Continuation Page for #5

APPLICATION / SUBMISSION INFORMATION

6. Type of Application/Submission Which This Certification Accompanies

☐ IND ☐ NDA ☐ ANDA ☐ BLA ☐ PMA ☐ HDE ☐ 510(k) ☐ PDP ☐ Other

7. Include IND/NDA/ANDA/BLA/PMA/HDE/510(k)/PDP/ Other Number *(If number previously assigned)*

If BLA was selected in item 6, provide Supplement Number

8. Serial Number Assigned to Application/Submission Which This Certification Accompanies

CERTIFICATION STATEMENT / INFORMATION

9. Check only one of the following boxes *(See instructions for additional information and explanation)*

☐ A. I certify that the requirements of 42 U.S.C. § 282(j), Section 402(j) of the Public Health Service Act do not apply because the application/submission which this certification accompanies does not reference any clinical trial.

☐ B. I certify that the requirements of 42 U.S.C. § 282(j), Section 402(j) of the Public Health Service Act do not apply to any clinical trial referenced in the application/submission which this certification accompanies.

☐ C. I certify that the requirements of 42 U.S.C. § 282(j), Section 402(j) of the Public Health Service Act apply to one or more of the clinical trials referenced in the application/submission which this certification accompanies and that those requirements have been met.

Certification Statement / Information section continued on page 2

FORM FDA 3674 (2/13) Page 1 of 2 PSC Publishing Services (301) 443-6740 EF

Figure 4.12 (a) FDA Form 3674—Certification of Compliance (1/2) and

CERTIFICATION STATEMENT / INFORMATION *(Continued)*

10. If you checked box C, in number 9, provide the National Clinical Trial (NCT) Number(s) for any "applicable clinical trial(s)," under 42 U.S.C. § 282(J)(1)(a)(i), section 402(j)(1)(a)(i) of the Public Health Service Act, referenced in the application/ submission which this Certification accompanies. *(Add continuation page as necessary.)*

NCT Number(s): ______ ______ ______ ______ ______

Continuation Page for #10

The undersigned declares, to the best of her/his knowledge, that this is an accurate, true, and complete submission of information. I understand that the failure to submit the certification required by 42 U.S.C. § 282(j)(5)(B), section 402(j)(5)(B) of the Public Health Service Act, and the knowing submission of a false certification under such section are prohibited acts under 21 U.S.C. § 331, section 301 of the Federal Food, Drug, and Cosmetic Act.

Warning: A willfully and knowingly false statement is a criminal offense, U.S. Code, title 18, section 1001.

11. Name and Title of the Person who Signs Number 15

Name	Title

12. Address

Address 1 *(Street address, P.O. box, company name c/o)*	
Address 2 *(Apartment, suite, unit, building, floor, etc.)*	
City	State/Province/Region
Country	ZIP or Postal Code

13. Telephone and Fax Numbers *(Include country code if applicable and area code)*

(Tel): ______

(Fax): ______

14. Date of Certification

15. Signature of Sponsor/Applicant/Submitter or an Authorized Representative *(Sign)*

Sign

This section applies only to requirements of the Paperwork Reduction Act of 1995.

*****DO NOT SEND YOUR COMPLETED FORM TO THE PRA STAFF EMAIL ADDRESS BELOW.*****

The burden time for this collection of information is estimated to average 15 minutes and 45 minutes (depending on the type of application/ submission) per response, including the time to review instructions, search existing data sources, gather and maintain the data needed and complete and review the collection of information. Send comments regarding this burden estimate or any other aspect of this information collection, including suggestions for reducing this burden to:

Department of Health and Human Services
Food and Drug Administration
Office of Chief Information Officer
Paperwork Reduction Act (PRA) Staff
PRAStaff@fda.hhs.gov

"An agency may not conduct or sponsor, and a person is not required to respond to, a collection of information unless it displays a currently valid OMB number."

FORM FDA 3674 (2/13) Page 2 of 2

Figure 4.12 Continued (b) FDA Form 3674—Certification of Compliance (2/2).

Table 4.9 Comparison of 510(k) and PMA submissions [117]

510(k)	PMA
Primarily for Class II devices (moderate risk)	Primarily for Class III devices (high risk)
A legally marketed "predicate" device exists	A Class I or II legally marketed predicate device does not exist
Documented proof of substantial equivalence to predicate device is required	Documented reasonable safety and effectiveness data for the device are required
	Device is life supporting or sustaining, of substantial importance in preventing impairment of human health, or can present a potential unreasonable risk of illness or injury

PMA contents and documents

Premarket approval (PMA), by FDA definition, is any premarket approval application for a Class III (high risk) medical device, including all information submitted or incorporated by reference [118]. Like the 510(k) submission, there is no fixed template for a PMA application. Furthermore, six copies of a PMA should be prepared and each bound with numbered volumes of reasonable size. Additional copies of the PMA should be provided upon request by the FDA and trade secret, confidential, commercial, and financial information must be included in all copies of the PMA, and identified in at least one of the copies. Required elements of a PMA application [119] are as follows:

General Requirements for PMA Submission (with reference to Table 4.10) *(1) Medical Device User Fee Cover Sheet [MDUFA PMA Cover Sheet]* A PMA submission must also be accompanied with a MDUFA PMA cover sheet, which can be found at the same FDA User Fee Web site [92] that generates the MDUFA 510(k) cover sheet. The FY15 User Fees (Table 4.14) [93] for a PMA submission is US$250,895. Payment of user fees must be done on or before the date of submission. Any application received without payment will be considered incomplete. For more detailed step-by-step instructions, please refer to the FDA User Fee Web site [92, 94].

(2) PMA Cover Letter [119] ——————————— **Template for PMA Cover Letter (Start)**

Original PMA Cover Letter

[Date]

PMA Document Mail Center - WO66-G609
Center for Devices and Radiological Health
Food and Drug Administration
10903 New Hampshire Avenue
Silver Spring, MD 20993-0002

SUBJECT: Original PMA for *[device trade name and model number if applicable]*

To Whom It May Concern:

Table 4.10 **Required elements for PMA**

1	MDUFA Cover Sheet	Cover Sheet generated at FDA User Fee Web site
2	Cover Letter	Format provided
3	Applicant Details	Name and address
4	Table of Contents	Specify volume and page number for each item in table • Separate sections for nonclinical laboratory studies and clinical investigations involving human subjects
5	Summary Section	• Indications for use • Device description • Alternative practices and procedures • Marketing history • Summary of studies • Conclusions
6	Complete Device Description	• Device components • Properties of device relevant to treatment/diagnosis • Device operation • Manufacturing process
7	Reference to Standard	• Performance standard • Established under RCHSA (21 CFR 1000-1050) • Voluntary standard • FDA recognized consensus standards
8	Technical Data and Information	• Result of nonclinical laboratory studies • Result of clinical investigations involving human subjects
9	Justification	• If PMA supported by data from only one investigation, justification must be provided
10	Bibliography of Published Reports	• Copy of key articles/data/information/report, brief summary of prominent features of article and brief discussion of related safety and effectiveness evaluation should be provided
11	Device Sample	Sample of device and components should be submitted to FDA if requested. If not convenient, location of which device may be examined, should be provided
12	Proposed Labeling	Copies of all proposed labeling should be provided: • Instructions for installation • Advertisement, etc.
13	Environmental Assessment	Not ordinarily required. Refer to PMA Special Consideration section for more details
14	Financial Disclosure or Disclosure Statement	As required by 21 CFR 54
15	Other Information	Upon request

[Applicant's name] is submitting this original premarket approval application for the *[device trade name], [device generic name]* intended for use in *[indication for use]*.

Clinical studies of the above device were initiated on *[date]* and *[were/were not]* conducted under an approved investigational device exemption *[give IDE number if a significant risk device]*. [If applicable, include the FDA reference number for any premarket notification, reclassification petition, or color additive petition submitted for this device].

[Include a paragraph providing the name and address of each facility involved in the manufacture of the device and indicate whether the facility is prepared for an FDA inspection. If not prepared, provide an expected date when the facility will be ready for inspection. If a waiver of the QS information is requested, provide an anticipated date that the information will be provided.]

If another document is incorporated by reference, e.g., a master file, please include the original letter of authorization as an attachment to this cover letter.

The existence of this PMA and the data and other information that it contains are confidential, and the protection afforded to such confidential information by 18 USC 1905, 21 USC 331(j), 5 USC 552, and other applicable laws is hereby claimed. [Tip: confidentiality claims cannot be made unless the applicant has complied with the applicable requirements.

If there are questions regarding this submission, *[name]* may be contacted at *[give telephone number including area code]*.

Sincerely yours,

[signature]

[Name and title of applicant's representative]

Template for PMA Cover Letter (End)

(3) Applicant Details Full name and address of applicant must be provided. If applicant does not live in United States, or have a business within the United States, the information and details of the authorized representative who lives and maintains a business in the United States should be provided.

(4) Table of Contents The table of contents should clearly specify numbered volume and page numbers and include separate sections for nonclinical studies and clinical studies involving human subjects.

(5) Summary Section A summary of general understanding of the device should be provided. This includes the general purpose of the device and targeted patient population under "Indications for use," Basic "Device description," device proprietary/trade name, functions, scientific concepts, and manufacturing process. Any "Alternative practices and procedures" should be included with its "Marketing history" in foreign and US market if known, and a list of all countries in which the device has been marketed or withdrawn for any safety- or effectiveness-related reasons. "Summary of studies" must include study objective, experimental design, brief discussion of data collection and analysis, brief description of findings, and conclusions. The summary should also contain a summary of nonclinical laboratory studies and clinical investigations involving human subjects. The summary for clinical investigations should include subject selection and exclusion conditions, safety and effectiveness data, adverse reactions, complications, device failures, and any other information as appropriate. Any investigation conducted under an IDE must be identified. Discussion of how data and information in the application proves Safety and Effectiveness in 21 CFR 860.70 [120] will be done in "Conclusions drawn from the studies."

(6) Complete Device Description A complete device description should have:

- Device description with pictures and device components or ingredients (if applicable);
- Properties of device relevant to treatment, diagnosis, prevention, cure, or mitigation of a disease or condition;
- Principles of operation of device; and
- Sufficient details of methods, facilities, controls used in manufacturing, and installation process.

(7) Reference to Standards For reference made with any standards, adequate information should be provided to show how the device meets or deviates from the standard used. There are two types of standards referred to by the FDA. Performance standards are circulated under Part 514 of FD&C Act or the Radiation Control for Health and Safety Act of 1968 (RCHSA). At the moment, there is only one performance standard established for medical devices (21 CFR 898—Performance Standard for Electrode Lead Wires and Patient Cables) [121]. RCSHA performance standards are available on the Internet [122]. Another set of standards are voluntary standards, which are FDA recognized standards previously mentioned [113] and are specifically applicable to any aspect of safety or effectiveness of a device and developed according to the FDA.

(8) Technical Data and Information Adequate information and data should be provided for the FDA to determine whether to approve or reject the application. Information should include:

- Nonclinical laboratory studies (if applicable):
  - Microbiological
  - Toxicological
  - Immunological
  - Biocompatibility
  - Stress
  - Wear
  - Shelf life
  - Animal Studies

  A statement should be included that each study was conducted in compliance with Good Laboratory Practice for Nonclinical Laboratory Studies (21 CFR 58) [123]. If study was not conducted in compliance with 21 CFR 58, brief justification of noncompliance should be provided.
- Clinical investigation (involving human subject):
  - Protocols
  - Investigators and subject ratio with details

- Subject selection and exclusion criteria
- Study population demographics
- Study period
- Safety and effectiveness data with analysis and discussion of any impact
- Analysis and discussion of any potential biases related to gender, race/ethnicity, etc.
- Adverse reactions and complications
- Patient discontinuation/complaints
- Device failures/replacements
- Data tabulations of individual subject reporting forms
- Results of statistical analyses of clinical investigations
- Contraindications and precautions for use of device
- Other information, as appropriate

  Statements should be included with respect to each study:
  - That it either was conducted in compliance with 21 CFR 56—Institutional Review Boards or was not subject per 21 CFR 56.104—Exemptions from IRB Requirement or 21 CFR 56.105—Waiver of IRB Requirement [124]
  - That it was conducted in compliance with Subpart B of 21 CFR 50—Informed Consent of Human Subjects [125]
  - That it was conducted in compliance with 21 CFR 812—Investigational Device Exemptions [126] concerning sponsors of clinical investigations and clinical investigators

  If study was not conducted in compliance with these regulations, brief justification of noncompliance should be provided.

(9) Justification If a PMA is supported by data from only one investigator, justification is needed showing why data and other information from a single investigator is enough to prove safety and effectiveness of the device and to guarantee reproducible test results.

(10) Bibliography of Published Reports A copy of all the key articles, data and any known information, a brief summary of prominent features of the article, and a brief discussion of related safety and effectiveness evaluation should be provided.

(11) Device Sample One or more samples of the device and its components should be submitted if requested by FDA. If not practical to submit a device sample, location at which sample device may be examined and tested should be provided.

(12) Proposed Labeling Labeling must comply with 21 CFR 801—Labeling [110] and copies of all proposed labeling for the device should be submitted. Labeling must include:

- Common name of device
- Quantity of contents
- Name and address of manufacturer

Labeling may also include prescription use restrictions, information for use (indications for use, effects, routes, methods, frequency and duration of administration, relevant hazards, etc.) Indications for use are based on nonclinical and clinical studies described in the PMA [127].

(13) Environmental Assessment In accordance with 21 CFR 25—Environmental Impact Considerations [128], an Environmental Assessment (EA) should be included. For a device that is of the same type and same use as a previously approved device, the PMAs do not usually need an EA. For more exclusions, refer to 21 CFR 25.30 and 21 CFR 25.34.

(14) Financial Certification or Disclosure Statement The Financial Certification Form 3454 (Figure 4.8) or Disclosure Statement Form 3455 (Figure 4.9), the same as used in 510(k), or both as required by 21 CFR 54—Financial Disclosure by Clinical Investigators [129] should be provided.

(15) Other Information FDA will request other information if required.

PMA (IDE)

As quoted by the FDA, "Premarket approval (PMA) is the FDA process of scientific and regulatory review to evaluate the safety and effectiveness of Class III medical devices." Thus, prior to a PMA application, clinical studies are to be done in order to support the PMA and also provide evidence of safety and effectiveness of a medical device. Hence, an Investigational Device Exemption (IDE) must be applied to allow the investigational device to be used in a clinical study. This IDE application would also be relevant to 510(k)s that require clinical data. The IDE must be approved by an institutional review board (IRB), and the FDA if the study involves a significant risk device (which is determined during Presubmission of an IDE). Required elements of an IDE application (Table 4.11) and cover letter (Table 4.12) are shown [130]. The PMA submitter should also register their clinical studies at *ClinicalTrials.gov* [131] and submit results to aid the IRB to determine appropriateness of the study.

4.2.4 Step 4: Send premarket submission to FDA for review

After preparation of all relevant documents, submitter must first submit user fees before submitting any application to the FDA. If application is received without payment (either before or during submission), application is deemed incomplete and will not be reviewed or processed. Besides hardcopies, submissions must also include an electronic copy (eCopy) on a compact disc (CD), digital video disc (DVD), or a flash drive [132]. After submission, the FDA will conduct an Administrative Filing Review to check if the submission is sufficient to be reviewed. During review, the FDA staff will communicate through an Interactive Review to increase the efficiency of the review process (Table 4.13).

4.2.4.1 Submission fees and timeline

Table 4.13 shows the User Fees for Fiscal Year 2015 [93] and is usually paid in the form of a MDUFA Cover Sheet. All types of 510(k) are subjected to the same user fee; however, there is no user fee submitted to the FDA if submission is through an FDA-

Table 4.11 IDE required elements (in order)

1	Sponsor details	Name and address
2	Report of prior investigations of device for: • Clinical testing • Animal testing • Laboratory testing	Include: • Bibliography of publications adverse/supportive • Copies of all published/unpublished adverse information • Copies of other significant publications (if requested) • Summary of all other unpublished information relevant to safety and effectiveness evaluation of device • Statement for compliance/ incompliance with GLP with reason for the latter
3	Investigational plan	**1.** Purpose **2.** Protocol **3.** Risk Analysis **4.** Device Description **5.** Monitoring Procedures **6.** Additional Records and Reports
4	Description of manufacture process, packaging, storage, and installation:	• Methods • Facilities • Controls
5	Example of agreement (signed by investigators) with list of names and address of all investigators	
6	Certification for signing of agreement	
7	Contact list for IRB reviewers	
8	Other institution where part of investigation may be conducted	Name and address
9	Amount charged for device (if any)	
10	Labeling for device	Copies of all labeling
11	Consent forms	Copies of all informed consent forms (Protection of Human Subjects)
12	Other relevant information	Requested by FDA

accredited third party reviewer (as mentioned in Section 4.2.3.2.1 under MDUFA 510(k) Cover Sheet) [95] (Figure 4.13).

The 510(k)s are reviewed by staff consisting of a team of scientific professionals from the Office of Device Evaluation (ODE) and the Office of in vitro Diagnostics and Radiological Health (OIR), under the FDA's Center for Devices and Radiological Health (CDRH). The divisions are organized by medical device specialties.

Table 4.12 Suggested contents for original IDE application cover letter (in order)

(1)	Statement that information provided is an original IDE submission	
(2)	Device information	• Device name • Intended use
(3)	Sponsor information	• Name • Address[a] • Contact person • Telephone number • Fax • Email
(4)	Manufacturer information	• Name • Address • Contact person • Telephone number • Fax
(5)	Correspondent information	If organization submitting application is not sponsor, include contact information for correspondent organization or individual.
(6)	Other information (if applicable)	• Presubmission to FDA: State Pre-Sub number and a copy of written feedback • Presubmission meetings with FDA: State name of FDA contact person and a copy of meeting minutes
(7)	Waiver requests and justification	If applicable
(8)	Referenced files in IDE application	Example: • PMA • 510(k) • IDE

[a] Sponsor must be located in United States according to 21 CFR 812.18(a).

Table 4.13 FY15 User Fees (US$)

Submission type	Standard fee	Small business fee[a]
510(k)	$5,018	$2,509
PMA	$250,895	$62,724

[a] Small business fee is applicable for small businesses with gross sales of less than $30 million or that have an FDA approved SBD (Small Business Determination). Small businesses with approved SBD are also eligible to have their first PMA user fee waived [133].

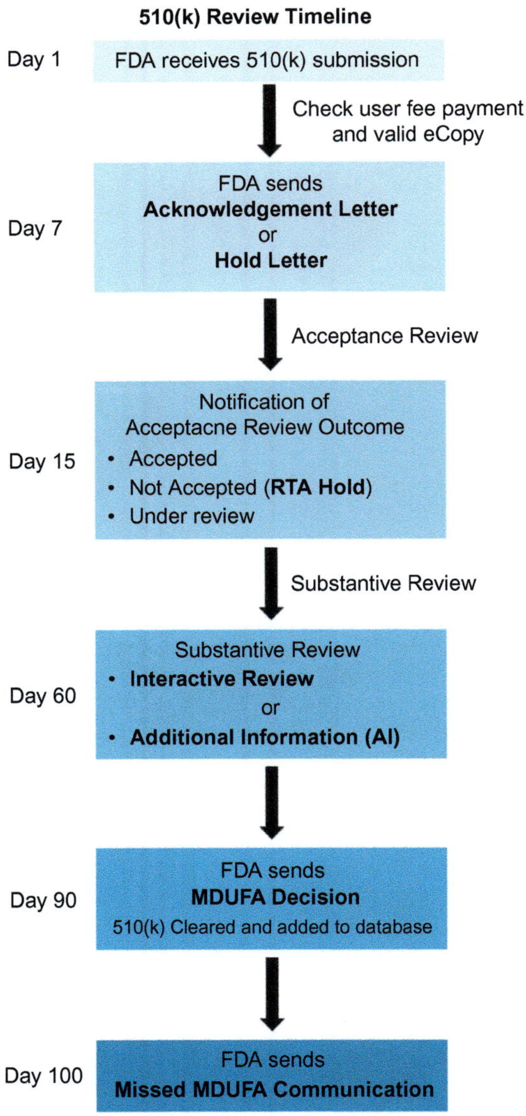

Figure 4.13 Timeline and General 510(k) Review Process. All days are calendar days.

When a 510(k) is received (Day 1), the Document Control Center (DCC) assigns a K or 510(k) number, which follows this submission throughout its entire lifetime. If the 510(k) is cleared and the device successfully marketed, the 510(k) then becomes its identity.

As shown in Figure 4.14, the 510(k) number consists of six numbers, the first two numbers being the year in which the 510(k) is received, and the last four are consecutive numbers as per number of submissions received by the FDA that year. For example, the first submission of 2015 would be K150001.

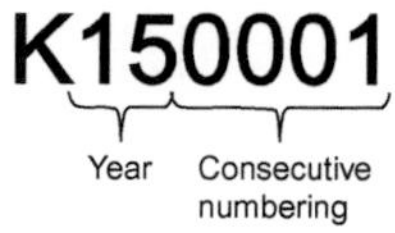

Figure 4.14 The 510(k) or K Number.

After a 510(k) number is assigned, the DCC then does a check for user fee payment and valid eCopy. By Day 7 (from when the submission is first received), the FDA sends either an Acknowledgment Letter (if user fee has been paid and/or with valid eCopy submitted) or a Hold Letter (if the user fee and eCopy are not in order).

Once the 510(k) submission passes the check, the FDA will proceed with an Acceptance Review to check if the 510(k) documents are acceptable for Substantive Review, and sends an electronic notification by Day 15 to notify that submissions is either Accepted for Substantive Review, Not Accepted (Refuse to Accept, RTA Hold), or under review if the FDA did not complete the acceptance review in 15 days. If an RTA Hold is not fully addressed within 180 days, a new 510(k) for the same device will need to be submitted as the 510(k) submitted previously will be considered withdrawn and deleted from the FDA review system.

After the 510(k) is accepted, the FDA will proceed with Substantive Review and by Day 60, the FDA will notify via email, that either they will proceed with an Interactive Review (by email or phone) to resolve any outstanding issues with submission that may be addressed within a set timeframe as gauged by the FDA or submission is placed on hold as Additional Information (AI) is required. The AI request must be addressed with valid eCopy and received by DCC within 180 days from AI request date. Otherwise, the 510(k) will be considered withdrawn and removed from the review system.

The FDA aims to make a MDUFA decision, in the form of a decision letter via email, for a 510(k) submission within 90 days from when a 510(k) is received, excluding days on hold. Cleared 510(k)s will be added to the 510(k) database on a weekly basis.

If a MDUFA decision was not made within 100 days, a Missed MDUFA Communication would be issued by the FDA; this is a written feedback to the submitter. The written feedback would include estimated completion date and the major unresolved review issues which have prevented the FDA from granting a final decision. These will be discussed in a meeting or teleconference [134].

The PMA review timeline is not as well-defined as the 510(k) review timeline and takes more than twice the duration of a 510(k) review process. Upon receiving a PMA submission (Day 1), the FDA begins to check if the submission documents are sufficient to proceed for further in-depth review in a process called Filing Review, which is equivalent to the Acceptance Review for the 510(k). By Day 45 of receiving the PMA submission, the FDA will notify the submitter of the Filing Review outcome and deficiencies (if any), with a PMA reference number and filing date, and whether the PMA has been filed or refused (see Figure 4.15). The FDA may refuse to file a PMA if:

- The PMA has insufficient information required according to FD&C Section 515(c)(1)(A to G)—Application for Premarket Approval [135];
- The PMA has insufficient information required according to 21 CFR 814.20—Premarket Approval Application [136] and inadequate justification for any item omission;
- Applicant has pending 510(k) for the same device and FDA has not determined that the device falls within the scope of the PMA under 21 CFR 814.1 [118];
- The PMA contains inaccurate facts; or
- The PMA does not have the statement of either Financial Certification or Financial disclosure under 21 CFR 54 [129].

If the PMA is refused, applicant may:

- Resubmit the PMA with additional information to comply with requirements overlooked with reference to the PMA number of original submission.
- Request an informal conference with the Director of ODE to review FDA's decision within 10 days of refusal to file notice receipt. The FDA will hold informal conference within 10 days after receiving request and make a decision to file/refuse within 5 days after informal conference.
  - Due to limited resources, applicant has to decide between an informal conference (where the decision not to file the application will be reviewed) and a meeting with ODE to discuss specific deficiencies and measures required to correct these deficiencies.

After successful PMA filing, the date of filing marks the first day of a 180-day timeframe in which an in-depth scientific, regulatory, and Quality System review by appropriate FDA staff is conducted. During this period, the FDA will notify the applicant through major/minor deficiency letters of any information required by the FDA to complete the review of the application. Within 100 days of the PMA filing, the applicant may request a Day-100 Meeting to discuss and review the status of the PMA application. The FDA may also subject the PMA to a Panel Review (Substantive Review), with an outside panel of experts (advisory committee), if appropriate. Throughout the panel review, the FDA will act as a middleman to communicate with the PMA applicant and the advisory committee in response to questions raised and to provide information. At any point in time, if the applicant supplies significant new data or information on his or her own initiative or at the FDA's request, the review period may be extended up to 180 days.

On a side note, Modular PMA may not be subjected to this same PMA timeline as it is permitted to be submitted in modules and reviewed independently. The FDA reviews a Modular PMA under a 90-day clock and communicates via deficiency letters and acceptance letters to notify submitters of any outstanding issues and issues resolved, respectively. Any amendments submitted to address deficiency letters must be made within 90-days of the letter and the FDA will review submitted amendments within a 90-day period, unless another amendment is submitted, which will again reset the 90-day clock [137].

4.2.5 Step 5: Complete establishment registration and device listing

The FDA requires all establishments/facilities and its manufactured medical devices to be registered and listed annually online at the Device Registration and Listing Module (DRLM) through the FURLS (FDA Unified Registration and Listing

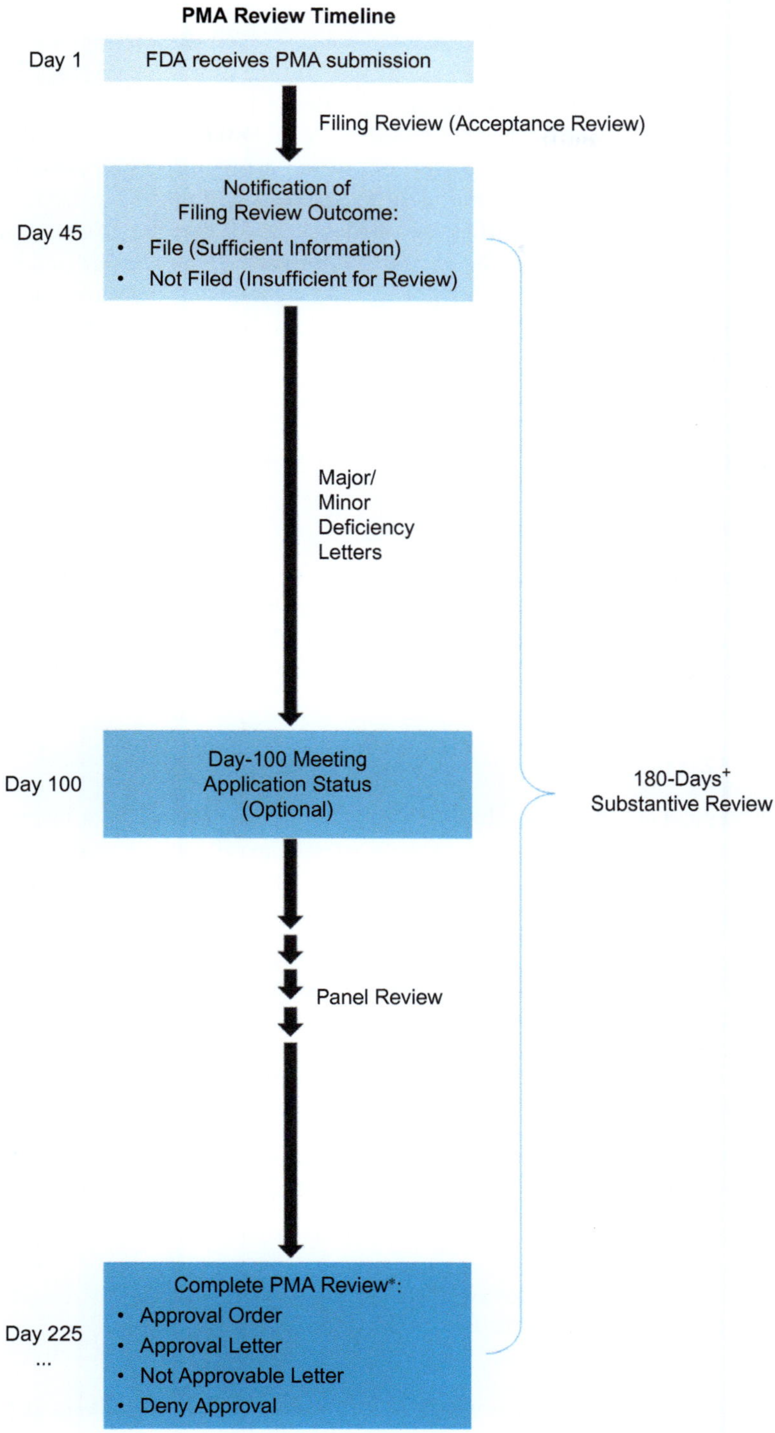

Figure 4.15 Timeline and general PMA review process.

System) Web site (https://www.access.fda.gov/oaa/) [138]. Before registration can be done, establishments are required to pay the user fee of US$3,646 (for FY15) at the Device Facility User Fee Web site [139], between 1st October and 31st December each year. After confirmation of payment, a PIN and Payment Confirmation Number (PCN) will be obtained for registration and listing in DRLM. Any changes in establishment/facility information and details may be updated in DRLM. The annual registration and listing will have to be done even if there are no changes. This is to make sure that establishment and device information are reviewed and kept up to date yearly. If a device is pending notification clearance or premarket approval, registration of establishment and listing will have to be done after the device has been cleared or approved.

4.3 European Union

4.3.1 The registration process

For manufacturers who intend to sell their medical devices in the EU market, the registration process is also the process to obtain the CE marking. According to 93/42/EEC, manufacturers should follow the procedures described in Figure 4.16. For Class I medical devices, the manufacturer may self-declare and affix the CE marking.

4.3.1.1 Class IIa and Class IIb

Class IIa medical devices, other than devices which are custom-made or intended for clinical investigations, the manufacturer shall, in order to affix the CE marking, follow the procedure relating to the EC declaration of conformity set out in Annex VII, coupled with either:

(a) The procedure relating to the EC verification set out in Annex IV; or
(b) The procedure relating to the EC declaration of conformity set out in Annex V (production quality assurance); or
(c) The procedure relating to the EC declaration of conformity set out in Annex VI (product quality assurance). Instead of applying these procedures, the manufacturers may also follow the procedure described under Class IIb medical devices (a).

Class IIb medical devices, other than devices which are custom-made or intended for clinical investigations, the manufacturer shall, in order to affix the CE marking, either:

(a) Follow the procedure relating to the EC declaration of conformity set out in Annex II (full quality assurance); in this case, point 4 of Annex II is not applicable; or
(b) Follow the procedure relating to the EC type-examination set out in Annex III, coupled with:
   (i) The procedure relating to the EC verification set out in Annex IV; or
   (ii) The procedure relating to the EC declaration of conformity set out in Annex V (production quality assurance); or
   (iii) The procedure relating to the EC declaration of conformity set out in Annex VI (product quality assurance).

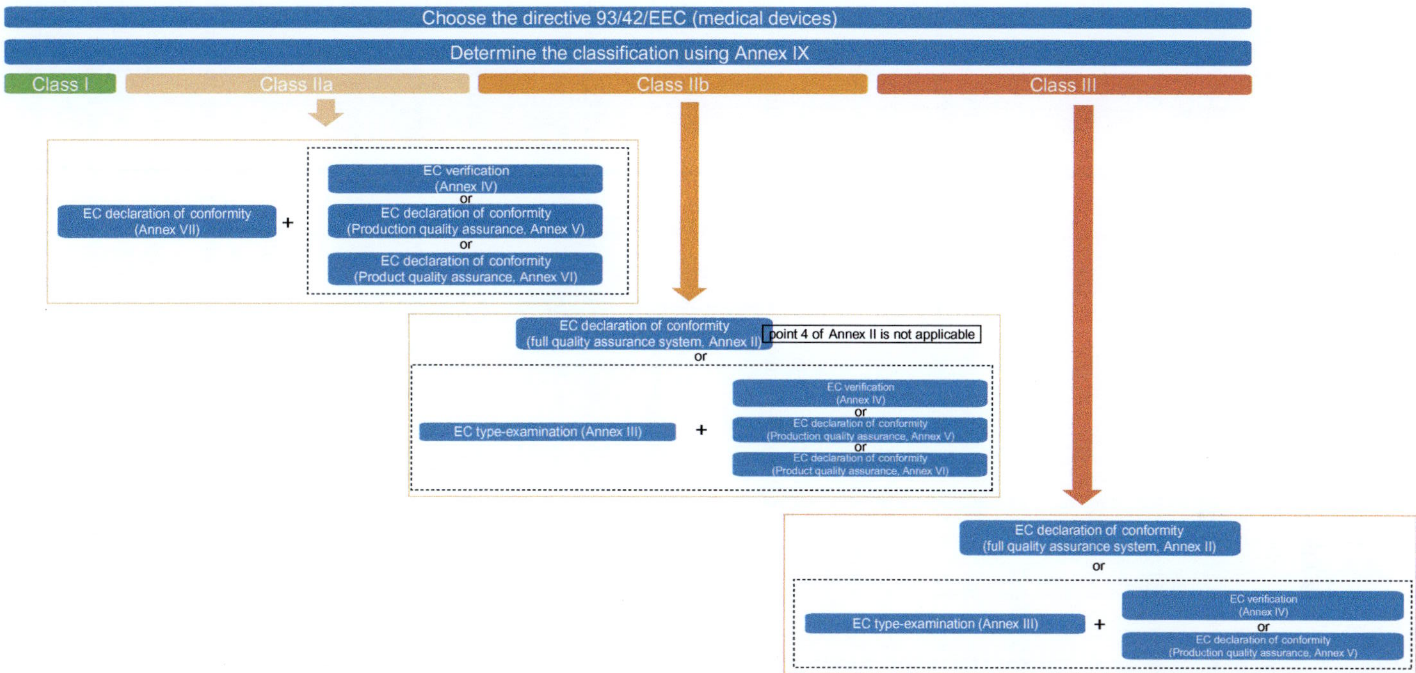

Figure 4.16 The procedure for medical device manufacturers who intend to obtain the CE marking to market their products in the EU.

4.3.1.2 Class III

Class III medical devices, other than devices which are custom-made or intended for clinical investigations, the manufacturer shall, in order to affix the CE marking, either:

(1) Follow the procedure relating to the EC declaration of conformity described in Section 4.3.2 (full quality assurance): or
(2) Follow the procedure relating to the EC type-examination set out in Annex III, coupled with:
   (i) The procedure relating to the EC verification set out in Annex IV; or
   (ii) The procedure relating to the EC declaration of conformity set out in Annex V (production quality assurance).

4.3.2 The required documents

The required documents for the medical device registration process (described in Section 4.3.1) are specified in Annex II–Annex VII of directive 93/42/EEC, and they are:

(1) Annex II: EC declaration of conformity (full quality assurance system);
(2) Annex III: EC type-examination;
(3) Annex IV: EC verification;
(4) Annex V: EC declaration of conformity (production quality assurance);
(5) Annex VI: EC declaration of conformity (product quality assurance); and
(6) Annex VII: EC declaration of conformity.

And the detailed information can be found in the directive 93/42/EEC, here we only give an example of Annex II: EC declaration of conformity (full quality assurance system).

This full quality assurance may apply for Class IIb and Class III. The manufacturer must lodge an application for assessment of its quality system with a notified body. The application must include:

(1) The name and address of the manufacturer and any additional manufacturing site covered by the quality system;
(2) All the relevant information on the product or product category covered by the procedure;
(3) A written declaration that no application has been lodged with any other notified body for the same product-related quality system;
(4) The documentation on the quality system;
(5) Confirmation that there is an undertaking by the manufacturer to fulfill the obligations imposed by the quality system approved;
(6) Confirmation that there is an undertaking by the manufacturer to keep the approved quality system adequate and efficacious; and
(7) Confirmation that there is an undertaking by the manufacturer to institute and keep up to date a systematic procedure to review experience gained from devices in the postproduction phase, including the provisions referred to in Annex X, and to implement appropriate means to apply any necessary corrective action. This undertaking must include an obligation for the manufacturer to notify the competent authorities of the following incidents immediately upon learning of them:

(i) Any malfunction or deterioration in the characteristics and/or performance of a device, as well as any inadequacy in the instructions for use which might lead to, or might have led to, the death of a patient or user or to a serious deterioration in his state of health;

(ii) Any technical or medical reason connected with the characteristics or performance of a device leading, for the reasons referred to in subparagraph (i), to systematic recall of devices of the same type by the manufacturer.

4.3.3 The turnaround time and fees

According to the statistics released by EMERGO, the time and fees for medical device registration in the EU are shown in Table 4.14 [140].

Table 4.14 Time and fees for medical device registration in EU [140]

Risk classification	Average timeline after submission until approval is granted	Overall cost of gaining regulatory approval
Class I nonsterile, nonmeasuring	<1 month	<US$5000
Class I sterile, measuring	3–5 month	US$15,000–30,000
Class IIa	3–5 month	US$15,000–30,000
Class IIb	3–6 month	US$30,000–50,000
Class III	6–9 month	US$30,000–50,000

Notes: The time frames shown in the table are typical for the majority of medical device submissions assuming that the device does not contain animal tissue or medicinal substances or employ entirely novel technology. The length of time to approval will depend on the quality and completeness of the technical documentation and how much time is taken to address additional information requests from authorities after submission. Submission(s) may take more time than what is shown.

4.4 China

4.4.1 The registration process

The general pathway for medical device registration in China is shown in Figure 4.17. The manufacturer needs to choose the right authority to submit the documents to depending on the classification of the medical device: domestic/import or Class II/Class III [141]. According to the new regulation and rules, registration is not required for Class I medical devices anymore; only filing is required [142].

4.4.1.1 Domestic Class II medical devices

The registration of domestic Class II medical devices consists of four main procedures, namely, submission, technical review, administration review, and approval and approval documents issuance [143]. For the submission, if the documents are

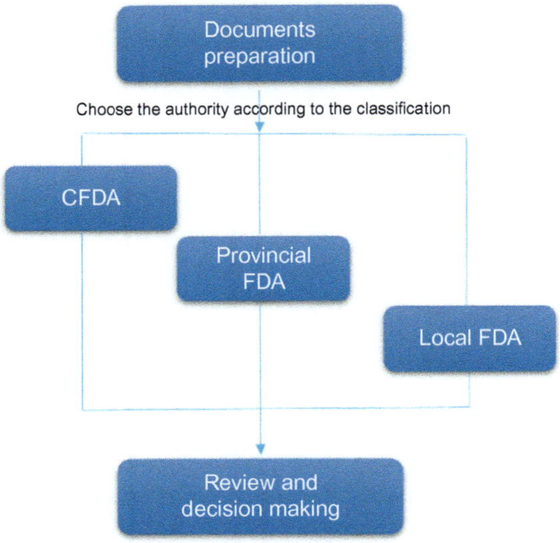

Figure 4.17 General pathway for medical device registration in China.

insufficient or fail to meet the requirements, the applicants should be informed within five working days. If the documents are qualified, the documents will proceed to be reviewed technically within three working days. The technical review will take 60 working days to complete. If any supplementary documents are required, applicant should provide the required documents within 1 year. Administrative review and approval will require 20 working days, and finally, the approval documents issuance requires another 10 working days. The whole process is shown in Figure 4.18.

The minimum duration for registration of domestic Class II is approximately 93 working days if all the necessary documents were sent in and qualified.

4.4.1.2 Domestic Class III and import Class II and III medical devices

The registration of domestic Class III and import Class II and III medical devices also includes four key procedures, and the key points are summarized as follows [144]:

- All documents (except certifying documents) must be written in Chinese.
- Chinese translation with endorsement is required for all certifying documents in foreign languages.
- All translated documents submitted must be submitted with original documents.
- Processing time is the same as for registration of domestic Class II devices.
- Technical review will take 60 to 90 working days.
- Administration review and approval will take 20 working days.
- Approval document issuance will take 10 working days.

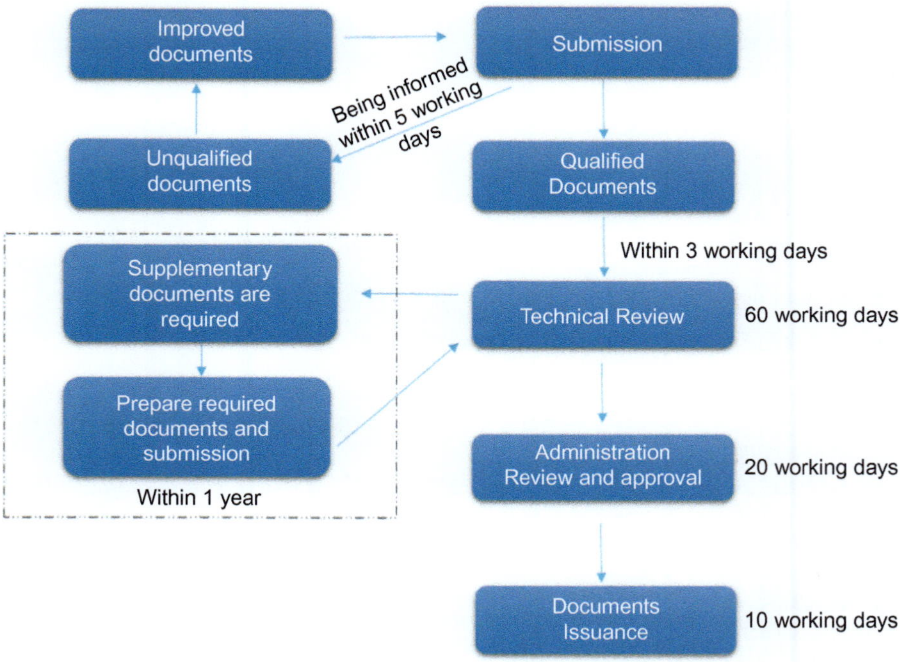

Figure 4.18 The registration process of domestic Class II medical devices in China.

4.4.2 The required documents

For registration of medical devices in China, the documents for registration or filing should be written in Chinese, and the documents which are translated from a foreign language should be submitted together with the original documents [45]. For registration of domestic Class II medical devices, the required documents are subject to each provincial FDA. For registration of domestic Class III and import Class II and III medical devices, the documents must be submitted to the CFDA.

4.4.2.1 Domestic class III medical devices

For domestic Class III medical devices, the required documents are [145]:

(1) Registration form for domestic medical devices;
(2) Photocopy of business registration documents and licenses;
(3) Organization code certificate of the People's Republic of China;
(4) Submission of notice for application under "Local innovative medical devices," according to the "innovative medical device approval process special approval;"
(5) As per "innovative medical device approval process special approval" for "Local innovative medical devices," for samples that were manufactured by other firms, submission of licenses of the company that was commissioned to manufacture the products and a letter of authorization issued to the commissioned company;
(6) Checklist for basic safety and efficiency requirement of medical device;

(7) Literature review;
(8) All research data;
(9) Manufacture and production information;
(10) Clinical evaluation data;
(11) Product risk assessment data;
(12) Product technical requirements;
(13) Product inspection report;
(14) Product manual and label design; and
(15) Declaration of conformity and checklist of conformity to standards.

The original documents are in Chinese, and the required documents are:

(1) 国家食品药品监督管理总局境内医疗器械注册申请表
(2) 企业营业执照副本复印件
(3) 组织机构代码证复印件
(4) 按照创新医疗器械特别审批程序审批的境内医疗器械提交创新医疗器械特别审批申请审查通知单
(5) 按照创新医疗器械特别审批程序审批的境内医疗器械,样品委托其他企业生产的,应当提供受托企业生产许可证和委托协议
(6) 医疗器械安全有效基本要求清单
(7) 综述资料
(8) 研究资料
(9) 生产制造信息
(10) 临床评价资料
(11) 产品风险分析资料
(12) 产品技术要求
(13) 产品注册检验报告
(14) 产品说明书及最小销售单元的标签设计样稿
(15) 符合性声明和符合标准的清单

4.4.2.2 Import Class II and III medical devices

The import medical devices should have been approved for marketing in the manufacturing country or territory [45]. The required documents are [146]:

(1) Registration form for import of medical devices;
(2) Document of proof for medical device to be marketed issued by medical device regulatory authority in the country of origin;
(3) Letter of authority issued by foreign applicant to the sole distributor in China;
(4) Letter of commitment by distributor(s);
(5) Copy of distributor's business license or copy of organization registration certificate;
(6) Checklist for basic safety and efficiency requirement of medical device;
(7) Literature review;
(8) Research data;
(9) Manufacture and production information;
(10) Clinical evaluation data;
(11) Product risk assessment data;
(12) Product technical requirements;
(13) Product inspection report;
(14) Product manual and label design;

(15) Declaration of conformity and checklist of conformity to standards; and
(16) Notarized document or original/English documents issued by the notary public.

The original documents are in Chinese, and the required documents are:

(1) 国家食品药品监督管理总局进口医疗器械注册申请表
(2) 境外申请人注册地或生产地址所在国家(地区)医疗器械主管部门出具的允许产品上市销售的证明文
(3) 境外申请人在中国境内指定代理人的委托书
(4) 代理人承诺书
(5) 代理人营业执照副本或者机构登记证明复印件综述资料
(6) 医疗器械安全有效基本要求清单
(7) 综述资料
(8) 研究资料
(9) 生产制造信息
(10) 临床评价资料
(11) 产品风险分析资料
(12) 产品技术要求
(13) 产品注册检验报告
(14) 产品说明书及最小销售单元的标签设计样稿
(15) 符合性声明和符合标准的清单
(16) 申请人所在地公证机构出具的关于原文/英文资料公证件

4.4.3 The turnaround time and fees

According to the normative documents released by the CFDA in 2014, the turn-around-time and fees are summarized in Table 4.15.

Table 4.15 Time and fees for medical devices registration in China

Risk classification	TAT for registration (working days)	Fees
Domestic Class II	93	Required, to be announced
Import Class II	123	Required, to be announced
Domestic Class III	93	Required, to be announced
Import Class III	123	Required, to be announced

Notes: the turn-around-time should be the minimum time the manufacturer expects. If any supplementary documents are required by the CFDA during the application, the actual time will be subject to the resubmission. For example, if external experts are required for the technical review, or the medical device–drug combination products require a more complex technical review, the turn-around-time will be longer than that mentioned in this table. But the technical review organization should inform the applicant about the turn-around-time in an official document [45].

4.5 Singapore

In Singapore, Class A nonsterile medical devices are exempted from product registration. Production registration for low-risk devices is required for Class A sterile medical devices, while product registration (CSDT dossier submission) is required for Class B, C, and D medical devices.

In Singapore, the HSA issued a guidance document: GN-22: Guidance for Dealers on Class A Medical Devices Exempted from Product Registration.

4.5.1 *The registration process*

The simplified process for medical device registration in Singapore [147] can be described as in Figure 4.19.

4.5.2 *The required documents*

4.5.2.1 *ASEAN Common Submission Dossier Template*

The Common Submission Dossier Template (CSDT) provides a common template for the submission of medical device information to medical device regulatory authorities of ASEAN member countries. In Singapore, the HAS issued the guidance documents: GN-17 Guidance on Preparation of a Product Registration Submission for General Medical Devices using the ASEAN CSDT [148, 149].

An executive summary shall be provided with the CSDT, which shall include the following information:

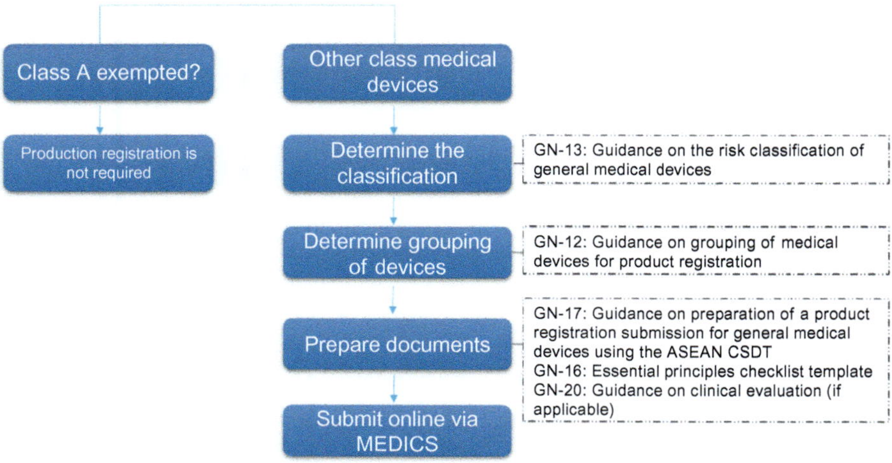

Figure 4.19 The medical device registration process in Singapore.

(1) An overview, e.g., introductory descriptive information on the medical device, the intended uses and indications for use of the medical device, any novel features, and a synopsis of the content of the CSDT;
(2) Commercial marketing history;
(3) Intended uses and indications in labeling;
(4) List of regulatory approval or marketing clearance obtained;
(5) Status of any pending request for market clearance; and
(6) Important safety/performance related information.

Elements of the CSDT include:

(1) Relevant essential principles and method used to demonstrate conformity;
- Essential principles and evidence of conformity;

(2) Device description;
- Device description and features;
- Intended use;
- Indications;
- Instructions for use;
- Contraindications;
- Warnings;
- Precautions;
- Potential adverse effects;
- Alternative therapy;
- Materials;
- Other relevant specifications; and
- Other descriptive information

(3) Summary of design verification and validation documents
- Preclinical studies: software verification and validation studies (if applicable); devices containing biological material
- Clinical evidence: use of existing bibliography;

(4) Device labeling;
- Samples of labels on the devices and its packing;
- Instructions for use;

(5) Risk analysis;
- Results of risk analysis; and

(6) Manufacturer information;
- Manufacturing process.

4.5.3 The turn-around-time and fees

The target turn-around-time for applications commences from the date of receipt of the application and does not include "stop-clock time" due to input requests for clarifications and additional information [150]. For medical device registration in Singapore, both application fees and evaluation fees are applicable. Evaluation fees are more expensive with higher risk. Additionally, annual retention fees for medical devices listed on the Singapore Medical Device Register (SMDR) are also required. From August 10, 2011, annual listing fees are payable for Class C and D medical devices; from January 1, 2013, annual listing fees are payable for Class A and B

Table 4.16 TAT and fees for medical devices registration in Singapore

Risk classification	TAT for registration	Application fees	Evaluation fees	Annual retention fee
Class A (sterile)	30	$25.00	–	S$25
Class B	60–160	$500.00	900–3500	S$35
Class C	120–220	$500.00	3000–5700	S$60
Class D	180–310	$500.00	5400–75,000	S$120

medical devices [151]. The turn-around-time and fees for medical device registration in Singapore are summarized in Table 4.16.

FAQs

(1) What is an eCopy and is there any format for an eCopy for premarket submission in the United States?

An eCopy, or Electronic Copy, is an exact duplicate of the paper submission, submitted together with the complete paper submission with a signed cover letter to the FDA. It can be submitted in the form of a compact disc (CD), digital video disc (DVD), or a flash drive. An eCopy is required for the following submissions:

- Premarket Notification (510k), including 510(k)s reviewed by third parties
- Premarket Approval (PMA)
- Investigational Device Exemption (IDE)
- *De novo* (Evaluation of automatic Class III designation petitions)
- Product Development Protocols (PDPs)
- Humanitarian Device Exemption (HDE), etc.

For format, waivers, exemptions, and other information, please refer to FDA guidance: eCopy Program for Medical Devices Submissions (http://www.fda.gov/downloads/MedicalDevices/DeviceRegulationandGuidance/GuidanceDocuments/UCM313794.pdf).

(2) What happens if an Abbreviated 510(k) or Special 510(k) cannot be reviewed as submitted?

If an Abbreviated 510(k) or Special 510(k) submitted is not eligible to be reviewed as submitted, reviewer will send notification of this issue and offer the option to either convert submission to a Traditional 510(k) or withdraw submission to be replaced with a future submission. If converted, the original receipt date remains as the start of the review period. Please note that additional information will be required for converted submission.

(3) Who are Accredited Third Parties? Can Accredited Third Parties review Abbreviated 510(k)s and Special 510(k)s? Are there any differences in fees and review time for submitting to a third party?

Accredited Persons, also known as accredited third parties, are people that are authorized by the FDA to conduct a primary review of 510(k)s for eligible devices. This Accredited Persons Program was created by the FDA Modernization Act of 1997 (FDAMA), based on an FDA pilot. For more information, please refer to FDA guidance "Implementation of Third Party Programs under the FDA Modernization Act of 1997; Final Guidance for Staff, Industry and Third Parties."

Accredited Third Parties may review both Abbreviated and Special 510(k) as long as the device to be reviewed is in the List of Eligible Devices for Third Party Review and User Fees to FDA are exempted as third parties generally charge for their services. The fees paid for a third party review is decided by an agreement between the 510(k) submitter and the accredited person, and price quotes from more than one third party may be obtained for comparison. The timeline for review is usually discussed before contracting for a review. If submission is done via a third party review, an authorization letter for the accredited person to discuss the 510(k) submission with the FDA on your behalf should be submitted.

(4) How long will it take for medical device registration in China?

The duration is subject to the classification of the medical device. For domestic Class II and III medical devices, the minimum time is 93 working days. For import Class II and III medical devices, the minimum time is 123 working days.

(5) What is a common submission dossier template (CSDT)?

A CSDT provides a common template for the submission of medical device information to medical device regulatory authorities of ASEAN member countries.

Part Two

Meeting regulations and standards

Risk assessment management for a new medical device

5

5.1 Introduction

Safety of a medical device is of the highest priority for any regulatory body and is the basis for product categorization and control. While a medical device being safe is the desired outcome, definition of what constitutes safe, and the procedures and actions to ensure safety require analyzing risk and its management. Thus identification and management of risk is a vital component in meeting regulatory requirements. European Council Directive 93.42.EEC on Medical Devices, ANNEX I Essential Requirements has safety as its first requirement followed by risk management as the second requirement as given in Table 5.1. Safety and risk arising from the various stages of the product's life cycle is not just limited to medical device regulations but may also be required from other related regulations such as environment and electronic devices.

Proper risk management goes beyond meeting regulatory requirements; it also includes ensuring the viability of the business. Safety related issues resulting in product recalls and liabilities (e.g., lawsuits) can be very costly and are often due to inadequate risk assessment. Risk assessment will help to define requirements along the product's life cycle and the corresponding tests to ensure product safety. Having clearance for sale of a medical device product by the regulatory body does not shield the manufacturer or product owner from responsibility in the event of injuries or death due its usage. However, risk assessment may protect the manufacturer or owner from liabilities if the hazards have been identified, mitigated, and conform to relevant safety standards such as ISO 10993 and IEC 60601.

Risk assessment is about balancing the product's benefit against risk. Such benefit–risk consideration may also influence the chosen path for medical device regulatory approval. Many invasive medical devices are high risk and may result in death in the event of device failure. However, without considering the benefits, the patient's life may be in greater danger or the quality of life may be very much reduced if the decision is based on risk alone. With proper risk assessment, peripheral risks may be significantly reduced such that the only major risk concern comes from just a few components and greater effort and resources may be used in mitigating them. To achieve this, a risk management plan is required.

Risk management is an on-going process and it goes beyond product introduction to the market. Thus, a risk management plan needs to be in place to ensure that risks throughout the product's life cycle are addressed. While most risk assessment is often associated with product design and development, it just covers part of the stages in a

Medical devices. http://dx.doi.org/10.1016/B978-0-08-100289-6.00005-3

Table 5.1 Extracts from the European Council Directive 93.42.EEC on medical devices, ANNEX I essential requirements

Clause 1	The devices must be designed and manufactured in such a way that, when used under the conditions and for the purposes intended, they will not compromise the clinical condition or the safety of patients, or the safety and health of users or, where applicable, other persons, provided that any risks which may be associated with their use constitute acceptable risks when weighed against the benefits to the patient and are compatible with a high level of protection of health and safety.
Clause 2	The solutions adopted by the manufacturer for the design and construction of the devices must conform to safety principles, taking account of the generally acknowledged state of the art. In selecting the most appropriate solutions, the manufacturer must apply the following principles in the following order: • eliminate or reduce risks as far as possible (inherently safe design and construction), • where appropriate take adequate protection measures including alarms if necessary, in relation to risks that cannot be eliminated, inform users of the residual.

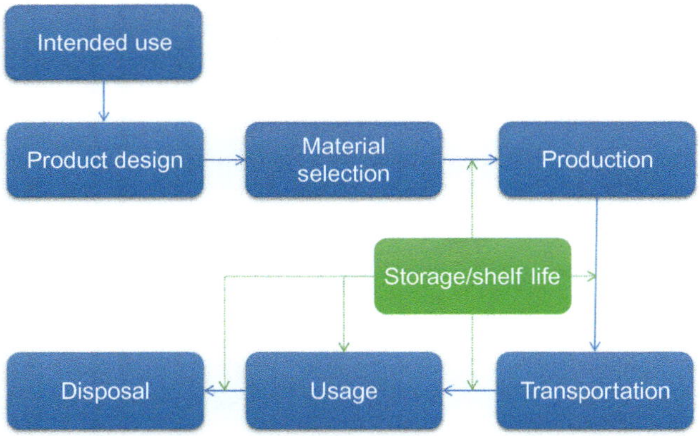

Figure 5.1 Example of a product life-cycle. Whether there are any risks at each stage is dependent on the product.

product life cycle as shown in Figure 5.1. Medical device regulations typically require risk assessment and control beyond product design. The European Council Directive 93.42.EEC on Medical Devices, ANNEX I Essential Requirements Clause 7.2 states that, "The devices must be designed, manufactured and packed in such a way as to minimize the risk posed by contaminants and residues to the persons involved in the transport, storage and use of the devices and to the patients ...." Therefore, it is just as important to look into material selections, production, transportation, storage, and the use of a device during risk assessment.

With a risk management plan, the associated documents on the risk assessment and report shall be constantly updated to reflect the stages in the product's life cycle. At the beginning stage of the product development, a preliminary risk assessment may be carried out based on the intended use of the product. This is usually a high level risk assessment to determine the foreseeable risk in the event of the product's failure to meet its intended use. This will also facilitate the classification of the product under the various regulatory bodies. Risk assessment across the various stages often requires the input from various stakeholders across various functional groups. To achieve this, a risk management system needs to be in place to guide the planning and designation of responsibilities. An example of the departments that may participate in the stages of a product's life cycle is shown in Table 5.2. Establishment of the system may be based on recognized international standards and guidelines on risk management.

National regulatory bodies often used recognized international standards or issue guidelines for risk management compliance. A general guideline recognized by the FDA, the European Commission (CE Mark), and major national regulatory bodies is the ISO 14971. The FDA also issues supplementary guidelines such as *Incorporating human factors into risk management* for product owners and manufacturers. Since most manufacturers typically use ISO 14971 to formalize a system for risk management, this shall be the framework for discussing risk management in this chapter.

Throughout the product's life cycle, from its development stage until its end-of-life, hazards and risks associated with it need to be identified and monitored to prevent recurrence. When failure occurs, analysis and correction must be fed back to the risk management process. This requires commitment and contribution across multiple departments and proper assignment of roles and responsibilities. Commitment from the senior management in the risk management process is crucial for provision of adequate resources and assignment of responsibilities. The senior management also needs to define risk acceptability, continuously review the adequacy of the risk management process due to changes or introduction of processes and changes to national regulations and international standards. A management representative is traditionally assigned to ensure compliance and execution of the management decisions. Documents are typically signed off by the management representative to indicate acceptance of the plan or results. This ensures accountability and commitment by senior management.

Table 5.2 Examples of product life cycle and relevant departments

Stages of product life cycle	Department
Product design	Research and Development, Quality Control, Manufacturing
Material selection	Research and Development, Procurement, Quality Control
Production	Manufacturing, Procurement, Logistic, Quality Control
Transportation	Logistic
Usage	Customer Service, Technical Support

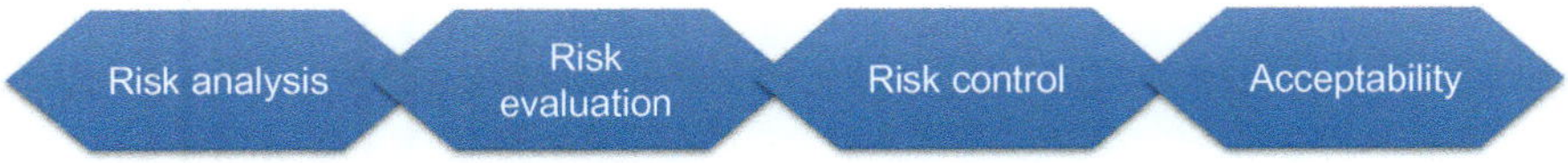

Figure 5.2 Key stages in risk management.

A risk management plan is needed to document the assignment of roles and responsibilities, provide an outline of the expected activities throughout the product's life cycle pertaining to risk management and the criteria for risk acceptability. A proper risk management plan will allow various departments to understand their role and what is expected of them in the risk management process of the particular product. As per ISO 14971, the risk management plan need not be complete at the beginning of the product development. It is expected that downstream risk associated with the product cannot be anticipated at the initial stages due to uncertainty in final product design, production model, distribution channels, and other things which will affect the risk management process. Thus, periodic review of the risk management plan is necessary in accordance with the product development and business decision.

Regardless of the product development stages and life cycle, the risk management process can be broken down into a few key stages as shown in Figure 5.2 with each part of the process building upon the earlier parts. As with the risk management plan, the risk analysis is expected to change throughout the product development and may be updated due to postproduction feedback, changes in regulatory requirement, or new information on hazards and risk related to the product.

5.2 Risk analysis

Risk analysis typically starts with identifying possible hazards associated with the product. A hazard is a high level categorization which leads to the identification of a hazardous situation. Examples of hazards are energy hazards, biological hazards, operational hazards, and information hazards. These hazards may be subdivided into lower level hazards such as electrical hazards, functional hazards, and labeling hazards. A hazard on its own may not cause harm to people or property. It is the presence of a hazard followed by a series of events that leads to a hazardous situation which causes harm. For example, although electrical energy is a hazard, it will only lead to a hazardous situation when its insulation is exposed or if the insulation is inadequate. From the risk analysis perspective, it is the hazardous situation that needs to be identified and addressed using various risk analysis techniques. The following are a few methods or sources for hazard and hazardous situation identification.

- **(a)** List of questions [77] [ISO 14971:2007 Annex C]
- **(b)** List of hazards categories. See Table 5.3
- **(c)** Speaking to experts, department/section representatives, users
- **(d)** Brain storming
- **(e)** Specific standards, guidance documents, regulatory requirements (e.g., IEC 60601)
- **(f)** Reported incidents on a regulatory site

Table 5.3 Examples of hazards [ISO 14971:2007 Annex E]

Examples of energy hazards	Examples of biological and chemical hazards	Examples of operational hazards	Examples of informational hazards
Electromagnetic energy Line voltage Leakage current • Enclosure leakage current • Earth leakage current • Patient leakage current Electric fields Magnetic fields *Radiation energy* Ionizing radiation Nonionizing radiation *Thermal energy* High temperature Low temperature *Mechanical energy* Gravity • Falling • Suspended masses Vibration Stored energy Moving parts Torsion, shear, and tensile force Moving and positioning of patient	*Biological* Bacteria Viruses Other agents (e.g., prions) Re- or cross-infection *Chemical* Exposure of airways, tissues, environment, or property, e.g., to foreign materials: • Acids or alkalis • Residues • Contaminates • Additives or processing aids • Cleaning, disinfecting or testing agents • Degradation products • Medical gasses • Anesthetic products *Biocompatibility* Toxicity of chemical constituents, e.g.: • Allergenicity/ irritancy • Pyrogenicity	*Function* Incorrect or inappropriate output or functionality Incorrect measurement Erroneous data transfer Loss or deterioration of function *Use error* Attentional failure Memory failure Rule-based failure Knowledge-based failure Routine violation	*Labeling* Incomplete instructions for use Inadequate description of performance characteristics Inadequate specification of intended use Inadequate disclosure of limitations *Operating instructions* Inadequate specification of accessories to be used with the medical device Inadequate specification of preuse checks Over-complicated operating instructions *Warnings* Of side effects Of hazards likely with reuse of single-use medical devices *Specification of service and maintenance*

Continued

Table 5.3 Continued

Examples of energy hazards	Examples of biological and chemical hazards	Examples of operational hazards	Examples of informational hazards
Acoustic energy • Ultrasonic energy • Infrasound energy • Sound High pressure fluid injection			

For common medical devices or for a project team with experience in the medical device, it may be possible to identify a list of hazards for analysis. An alternate source of hazards identification may come from looking at standards, guidance documents, and reported incidents. Some documents such as the IEC 60601 "Medical electrical equipment" [152,153], the ISO 10993 "Biological evaluation of medical devices" [6], and their subparts provide comprehensive information that addresses risk associated with medical devices. In particular, part one of IEC 60601 contains requirements on protection against hazards associated with electrical, mechanical, radiation, temperature, constructions, systems, and others. Another good source of hazard identification is from reported incidents available on regulatory body websites such as the Manufacturer and User Facility Device Experience (MAUDE) database from the FDA. It contains a list of reported incidents associated with all registered devices submitted to the FDA by mandatory reports and voluntary reporters. Users may find a product class that matches their own product and check for any associated reported events. The reports include the event type (hazard), description of the event, and the result of the manufacturer's investigation which states the possible cause and follow up actions.

5.3 Risk analysis techniques

There are several commonly used risk analysis techniques each with its strengths and weaknesses. Examples of risk analysis include preliminary hazard analysis (PHA), fault tree analysis (FTA), failure mode and effect analysis (FMEA), and hazard and operability analysis (HAZOP). Two techniques will be discussed here to illustrate risk analysis based on a top-down system approach and a bottom-up approach.

5.3.1 Failure mode and effect analysis

FMEA is a bottom-up risk analysis technique and it is one of the most popular methods because of its relative simplicity. As the name suggests, it involves identifying possible failure modes; the effect of failure followed by analyzing the cause of the failure.

The FMEA form typically comprises of columns with the following basic sections,

- Potential hazard (failure mode)
- Potential harm of failure (effects)
- Severity
- Cause of failure
- Probability/occurrence
- Risk level or risk priority number (RPN)
- Risk corrective measures

A failure is an event in which the medical device and its components did not function as intended or may have resulted in a hazardous event. Some examples of failure modes are operation failure, materials failure, mechanical failure, electrical failure, and failure of indications. It is important to include and anticipate all possible failure modes such that corresponding effects and cause can be predicted for preventive measures to be taken.

Effects of a failure will help to determine the cost or severity of the failure. It is common to find a failure effect that is caused by one or more failure modes. Examples of failure effect are machine stalling, no power, delayed response, and output error. Knowing the effect will help to assign the severity of the effect. Generally, the lowest level is "negligible" meaning no harm or damage and "catastrophic" is the highest level meaning death or serious injuries. The number of intermediate levels is determined by the manufacturer or the organization although it is common to find a total of three to five levels.

Knowing the failure mode will also help to determine the potential cause of it. Causes of failures may be attributed to machines or humans. Cause of failure due to a machine may be inadequate strength, insufficient power, inappropriate insulation, and software code error. Cause of failure due to a human is usually associated with insufficient training or lack of instructions on the machine.

It is common at the start of a project that the failure probability is a prediction based on limited available information. Prediction may come from verification testing, databases of similar items, or estimates from experts. The failure probability may be adjusted later when more data is available from production or customer feedback. Probability of failure typically ranges from improbable to frequent with a total of four to five levels.

Risk level and RPN are generated from the combination of severity level and failure probability. Although the intention is the same, there is a slight difference in using risk level and RPN in the determination of risk acceptability. Risk level works by placing the assigned severity and probability level in a matrix as shown below (Table 5.4).

Acceptability of the risk for each combination of probability and severity level is based on the matrix which is defined by the organization. Some organizations include an "Undesirable" category in the matrix to indicate risk corrective measures is

Table 5.4 Risk acceptability evaluation based on risk level through a severity and probability matrix

			Severity level			
		Level	Negligible 1	Minor 2	Serious 3	Catastrophic 4
Probability	Frequent	4	Undesirable	Undesirable	Unacceptable	Unacceptable
	Occasional	3	Acceptable	Undesirable	Unacceptable	Unacceptable
	Remote	2	Acceptable	Acceptable	Undesirable	Undesirable
	Improbable	1	Acceptable	Acceptable	Acceptable	Acceptable

Table 5.5 Acceptability determined by the assignment of the RPN

Category	RPN range
Unacceptable	≥ 9
Undesirable	$5 \leq \text{RPN} < 9$
Acceptable	<5

required if the combination falls into that category. The RPN works by a numerical multiplication of the probability and severity level. Acceptability is determined by the assignment of the RPN according to each defined category (Table 5.5).

Risk level and RPN each have its benefits and weaknesses. Risk level allows the organization to determine acceptability based on their preferred weighting of the severity and the probability. RPN is a numerical number which gives equal weight to severity and probability unless the equation or assignment of the value is modified to reflect preference. However, RPN can be used to include other considerations to the risk analysis such as the inclusion of detectability of failure value to the analysis.

Additional categories may be incorporated to the basic FMEA to capture more details to suit the organization's need. It is common to see a process step, product function, or component listed in the first column and identifying the potential hazard in the second column. Effects of the failure may also be further refined to effects at the local level and at the system level. For example, a faulty resister in an electrical printed circuit board may cause a bulb to fuse at the local level. At the system level, the effect is that there is no power signal light. In the risk analysis for a medical device, an additional column for probability after risk control measures is added to determine the residual risk level. It is important to note that any risk control measures will only reduce the probability of failure but not its severity. Other variants of the FMEA include the addition of a column for likelihood of detection. To verify that risk control measures have been implemented and are effective, an implementation column and effectiveness column may be added to include document references. Documents pertaining to implementation are work instructions, quality control procedures, component requirement specifications, engineering change documents, operating manuals, and others. Effectiveness documents may include inspection documents, drawings, postproduction monitoring, vendor evaluation forms, component compliance certificates, and others.

When considering using the FMEA as the risk analysis tool, it is important to know its weakness. Although the FMEA works well with medical devices with relatively simple systems and few components where failure of an entire system is traceable to the elements, it becomes very tedious for complicated machines with multiple functions and modular systems. For example, a dental archwire comprises of a single material which relies on its mechanical properties to effect teeth movement based on its profile. However, a complicated system such as a robotic surgery arm contains multiple systems such as electronic components, mechanical components, software, and others. Just listing the components in a FMEA will run into many pages. Complications and misunderstandings may arise when multiple redundancies are built into the system and the assignment of a failure mode and its cause is difficult to define as the relationship and inter-dependency between the components may not be well defined in the FMEA. For such larger complicated systems, a FTA may be more appropriate.

5.3.2 Fault tree analysis

The FTA is a systematic top-down method which starts from an assumption of a system failure followed by identification of the modes of system or component behavior that has contributed to this failure. These modes of system or component are not confined to hardware or software but include other factors such as human factors or interaction. FTA is particularly useful when quantitative data on probability is available although qualitative analysis can also be performed. In either case, an FTA can pinpoint common factors or the factors that are the highest contributor of system failure. This is not as readily identifiable using other risk analysis techniques such as FMEA. Its visual representation of the causes of the failure allows easy identification of a single fault event (a single failure that triggers a complete system failure). Where quantitative data is available, the probability of failures can be anticipated through mathematical calculations.

The FTA is comprised of a top event and a series of symbols, events, and logic gates for the construction of the tree. Some of the symbols commonly used in an FTA are shown in Table 5.6. Refer to IEC 61025 [154] for more symbols used in an FTA.

For complicated systems, the FTA diagram may become very large when the system failure is at a very high level. For example, a top event such as "system no response" in an electrical device may be due to numerous causes. In the absence of software to track the FTA, it is more practical to consider intermediate undesirable events such as "input power cut" or "transformer failure." This also allows different functional teams to work on various aspects of the FTA before combining at a later stage. Figure 5.3 is an illustration of how an FTA diagram looks for an alarm-related harm to patient in a medical system [155].

Table 5.6 Common symbols used in FTA

Symbol	Name	Description
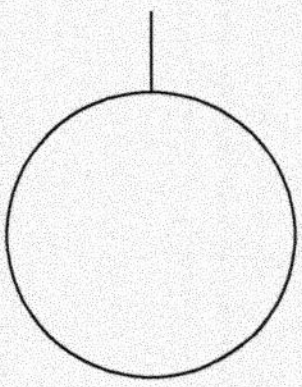	Basic event	Failure mode of a component or an individual failure cause
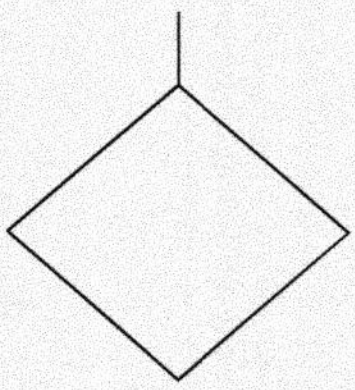	Undeveloped event	A potential failure mode or failure cause. However, relevant information is unavailable at the moment
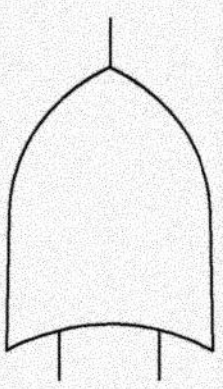	OR gate	Output event occur if any of the input events occur
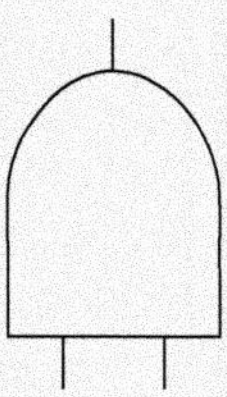	AND gate	Output event occur only if all the input events occur
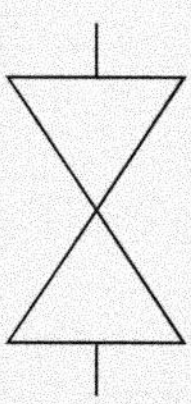	NOT gate	Output event occur only if all the input events DOES NOT occur

5.4 Application of risk analysis

Risk analysis is applied beyond the design and development stage. The same techniques may be used to perform risk assessment for other aspects of the product such as production, transport, usage, and disposal. While the main focus is on the product, it is also important to conduct risk assessment on auxiliary items such as labeling,

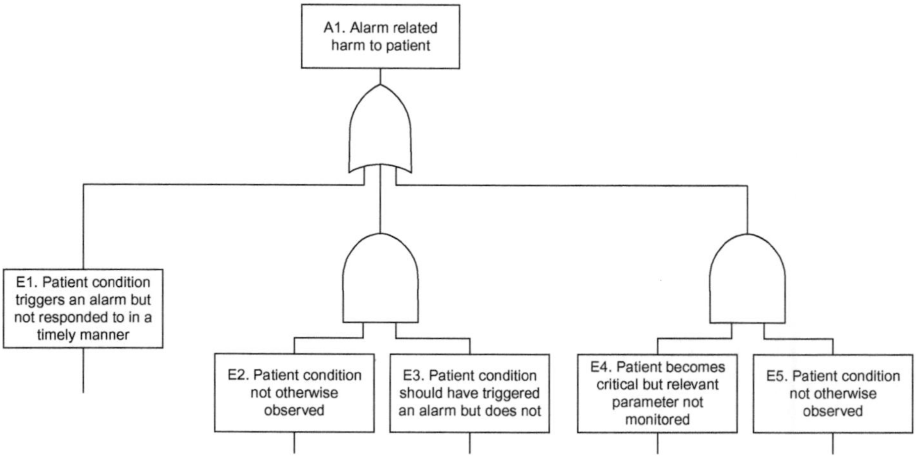

Figure 5.3 Illustration of FTA for alarm in a medical system [155].

packaging, and accompanying documents. For the FMEA, it is common to subdivide it into design FMEA (dFMEA), process FMEA (pFMEA), and application FMEA (aFMEA) as the column categories may be different for each of them. For an FTA, production issues, system issues, and user issues may also be included as the cause of an event failure. Figure 5.3 is an example of a medical system issue in a FTA of harm related to an alarm. Such harm can be caused by users not responding to the alarm or it could be due to product failure where the alarm is not triggered when it should have been.

5.5 Risk acceptability

There are several considerations for determining risk acceptability. Liability due to each risk needs to be considered. There is usually a cost involved in the reduction of the risk level for each failure mode. Risk reduction measures to meet an acceptable risk level will mean additional time and resources are expended. The risk level matrix as shown in Table 5.4 allows the management to communicate to the project team about their risk acceptability and actions to be taken for each risk level.

As required by ISO 14971, a risk/benefit analysis needs to be carried out if the risk is still not acceptable once all practicable risk reduction measures have been carried out. This is necessary to evaluate whether the benefits outweigh the harm. Generally, a design that is unacceptable will be abandoned. To justify that the benefits outweigh the harm such that the residual risk is acceptable is not a trivial affair. Sufficient evidence and extensive reviews and consultations need to be sought for this purpose. Evidence may come from clinical trials, or through in vitro and in vivo performance. Reviews and consultations in relation to alternative options and anticipated benefits need to be considered.

A person qualified because of his/her specialization, knowledge, and/or authority of the application will need to evaluate the overall residual risk.

5.6 Risk management report

The risk management report is a summary of the final results of the risk management process. Evidence of the implementation of the risk management plan needs to be included in the report. This may include references to the risk analysis documents. If a particular risk analysis method has been specified in the risk management plan, the document which records the risk analysis based on that method may be referenced. Any deviation from the risk management plan should be mentioned in the risk management report. It should also be indicated in the risk management report whether all the listed risks are acceptable. Where the overall residual risk exceeds the manufacturer's criteria for acceptable risk, the risk management report shall state its risk/benefit evaluation and determine whether the medical device should be marketed.

FAQs

(1) Why should a manufacturer perform risk assessment?

Risk assessment may protect the manufacturer or owner from liabilities if the hazards have been identified, mitigated, and conform to relevant safety standards such as ISO 10993 and IEC 60601.

(2) How does a national regulatory body determine the guidelines issued for risk management compliance?

National regulatory bodies often use recognized international standards or issue guidelines for risk management compliance. A general guideline recognized by the FDA, the European Commission (CE Mark), and major national regulatory bodies is the ISO 14971.

(3) Why are periodic reviews of the risk management plan necessary in accordance with the product development and business decision?

As per ISO 14971, the risk management plan need not be complete at the beginning of the product development. It is expected that downstream risk associated with the product cannot be anticipated at the initial stages due to uncertainty in final product design, production model, distribution channels, and other things which will affect the risk management process.

(4) What are some of the sources for hazards identification?

Some sources of hazards identification may come from looking at standards, guidance documents, and reported incidents such as IEC 60601 "Medical electrical equipment," ISO 10993 "Biological evaluation of medical devices," and their subparts which provide comprehensive information that addresses risk associated with medical devices. Another good source of hazard identification is reported incidents available on regulatory body websites such as the Manufacturer and User Facility Device Experience (MAUDE) database from FDA.

(5) What are some of the commonly used risk analysis techniques?

Examples of risk analysis include the Preliminary Hazard Analysis (PHA), the Fault Tree Analysis (FTA), the Failure mode and effect analysis (FMEA), and the Hazard and Operability Analysis (HAZOP).

(6) How is the acceptability of risk determined?

Acceptability of risk for each combination of probability and severity level is based on the matrix which is defined by the respective organizations.

(7) When should the FMEA be used as the risk analysis tool? Which risk analysis techniques is recommended for complicated machines with multiple functions and modular systems?

FMEA works well in medical devices with relatively simple systems and few components where failure of an entire system is traceable to the elements.

For larger and more complicated systems, a Fault Tree Analysis (FTA) may be more appropriate.

(8) What is the risk management report? What needs to be included?

The risk management report is a summary of the final results of the risk management process.

Examples of items to include in the risk management report are,

Things to include in Risk Management Report and its review

- Summary of risk Assessment method used Risk Assessment criteria
- Overall residual risk acceptability in particular cases where the risk item is acceptable due to its benefit over residual risk.
- Summary list of hazards that require further actions and their corresponding mitigation;
- Summary of changes to product design (if any). If there are any changes to product design, does it have any impact on its risk analysis?
- Are there any complain or incidents reported on our products that relates to its safety?
- Are there any feedbacks on our products along the value chain that relates to its safety?
- Are there any public reports, news or risk advisory on competitor's products or similar products? If there is, does it have an impact on our product's safety?
- Are there new regulatory guidelines regarding safety?
- Are there any updates on standards regarding safety?
- Review on Risk Assessment and highlight any important changes (if any) to the document.

Safety testing of a new medical device

6

6.1 Introduction

Safety of a medical device is the primary concern of any national regulatory organization. After the risks associated with the medical device have been considered, the next step is to carry out tests to ensure the safety of the product. The safety tests to be performed depend on numerous factors such as its intended use, packaging, whether it is sterilized, whether it is intended for one time use, and more. Safety of the device is not only restricted to the patient's safety, it also includes safety of the operators and anybody who may come into contact with the medical device. Related to the previous chapter of risk assessment, verification and validation of the product with regards to its safety needs to be performed once it is manufactured and ready to leave the production floor. Besides biocompatibility of the product, which needs to be considered where applicable, other safety considerations include packaging, transportation, and compatibility with other electrical appliances. It is important to appreciate that the range of medical products is huge with the FDA listing over 2000 devices spread over 19 medical specialties. This is not inclusive of medical devices that are not included in the list yet. It is not possible to come out with a complete list of safety tests to be performed given the diversity of medical products. The need for tests also depends on the risk analysis of the individual product. Figure 6.1 shows some general categories for safety tests.

Unlike performance and functional tests, safety tests are almost always based on established standards and procedures. Identification of the relevant standards is important to ensure that the design is compliant with regulatory requirements. Figure 6.2 gives an example of how this process can be carried out. The first step starts with knowing the intended use, the design, its components, and the product movement, people that come into contact with it and its life cycle. Because it is a medical device, the next step is to look at relevant medical device standards. These standards often reference other relevant standards that may or may not be specific to medical application. This will often provide sufficient coverage in terms of safety test requirements. There are numerous safety standards covering almost all conceivable designs, components, displays, labeling, and applications. Many of these standards are not written specifically for any medical device, however, your medical device or its component may still be covered by them depending on your design and intended use. Thus, for every design and component that has not been mentioned in the medical device standards, check whether there are any other related standards that could be applicable.

Each medical device is unique and is dependent on its design and intended use. This chapter will introduce some of the general major safety considerations for medical devices such as absence of toxic substance, biocompatibility, electrical safety,

Medical devices. http://dx.doi.org/10.1016/B978-0-08-100289-6.00006-5

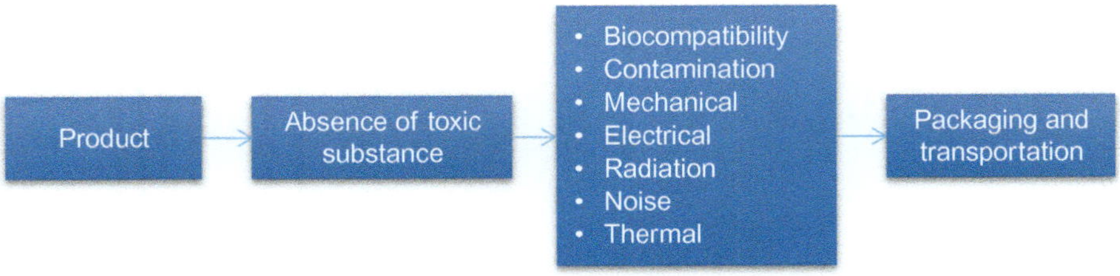

Figure 6.1 General categories for safety tests considerations.

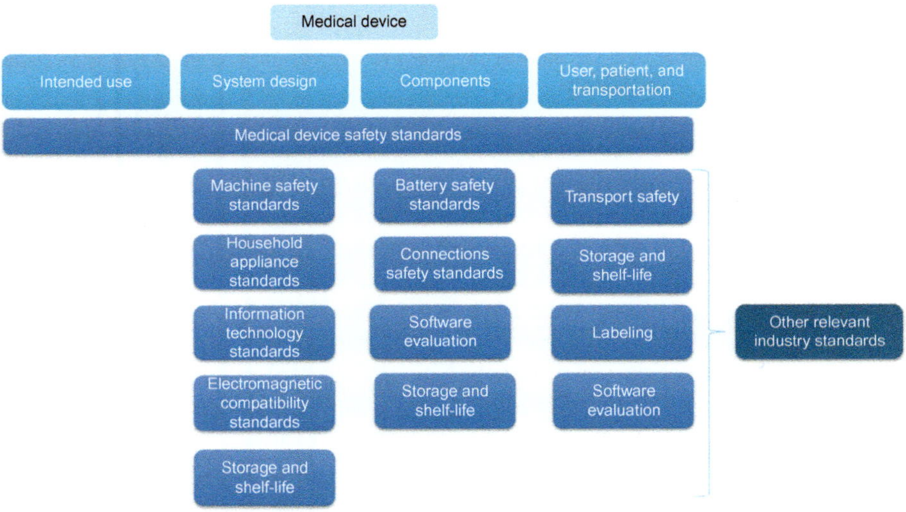

Figure 6.2 An example of how safety tests can be carried out.

mechanical safety, sterility, and transportation. Details of these tests and other tests that are more specific can be found in recognized standards and regulatory advisories.

6.2 Absence of toxic substance

The first consideration for any medical product is that it should be free from any toxic substance which may come from the material used, a coating, additives, or a sterilization process. Although there are many non-invasive medical devices or devices whose components may not come into contact with anybody, national regulatory bodies may still impose restriction on the presence of a toxic substance in products. Very often, a toxic substance may not come from the product itself but comes from the sterilization process before or between uses. For example, ethylene oxide (EO) is often used in sterilization and the level of EO residue poststerilization would need to be tested.

Table 6.1 Ref. Directive 2011/65/EU (restriction of the use of certain hazardous substances in electrical and electronic equipment)

Substance	Maximum concentration by weight (%)
Lead	0.1
Mercury	0.1
Cadmium	0.01
Hexavalent chromium	0.1
Polybrominated biphenyls (PBB)	0.1
Polybrominated diphenyl ethers (PBDE)	0.1

Electrical and electronic equipment marketed in the European Union, which includes electrical and electronic medical devices, needs to meet the requirement set up by Directive 2011/65/EU which is commonly known as restriction of the use of certain hazardous substances (ROHS). Under this directive, there are restrictions of certain substances and concentration limits as shown in Table 6.1.

Currently, there are no specific international test standards used for determining the concentration level of the toxic substance in a material. X-ray fluorescence (XRF) is often used for this purpose as it is nondestructive. A limitation of XRF is that it detects the elements but not the actual compound found in the material. Accuracy for lower end XRF is also probably insufficient to meet the concentration limits. More accurate techniques such as high performance liquid chromatography or gas chromatography/mass spectrometry may be used for the detection of chromium and bromine compounds. In any case, it is important to find out the detection limits of equipment used to test for concentration of the toxic substance. Proper calibration and records of the equipment accuracy is necessary for acceptance of test results.

Most electrical and electronic equipment contains numerous parts and components and each of these parts needs to be free of the specified toxic substance for the whole device to be ROHS compliant. Because it is not feasible or economical for the manufacturer to check each part for toxic substances, the alternative is to source for parts that are already ROHS compliant.

6.3 Biocompatibility tests

Biocompatibility tests are necessary for medical devices that come into contact with the patient. ISO 10993 Biological evaluation of medical devices are recognized by most major national regulatory bodies including the FDA and CE mark as the standard for selecting the biological tests necessary for assessing the safety of a medical device. Manufacturers need to determine which tests need to be performed and this depends on how the medical device is intended to be used. To facilitate manufacturers in determining the tests to be performed, ISO 10993-1 has listed the tests to be performed based on the area of contact between the medical device and the patient and its duration of contact as shown in Tables 6.2 and 6.3.

Table 6.2 Initial evaluation test for consideration

Nature of body contact			Biological effect					
Category	Contact	Contact duration A—Limited <24 h B—Prolonged 24 h to 30 days C—Permanent >30 days	Cytotoxicity	Sensitization	Irritation or intracutaneous reactivity	Systematic/ acute toxicity	Subacute and subchronic toxicity	Genotoxicity
Surface device	Skin	A	X	X	X			
		B	X	X	X			
		C	X	X	X			
	Mucosal membrane	A	X	X	X			
		B	X	X	X			
		C	X	X	X		X	X
	Breached or compromised surface	A	X	X	X			
		B	X	X	X			
		C	X	X	X		X	X
External communicating device	Blood path, indirect	A	X	X	X	X		
		B	X	X	X	X		
		C	X	X		X	X	X
	Tissue/bone/ dentin	A	X	X	X			
		B	X	X	X	X	X	X
		C	X	X	X	X	X	X
	Circulating blood	A	X	X	X	X		
		B	X	X	X	X	X	X
		C	X	X	X	X	X	X
Implant device	Tissue/bone	A	X	X	X			
		B	X	X	X	X	X	X
		C	X	X	X	X	X	X
	Blood	A	X	X	X	X	X	
		B	X	X	X	X	X	X
		C	X	X	X	X	X	X

Table 6.3 Supplementary evaluation test for consideration

Nature of body contact			Biological effect					
Category	Contact	Contact duration A—limited <24 h B—Prolonged 24 h to 30 days C—Permanent >30 days	Implantation	Hemocompatibility	Chronic toxicity	Carcinogenicity	Reproductive/development	Biodegradation
Surface device	Skin	A						
		B						
		C						
	Mucosal membrane	A						
		B						
		C						
	Breached or compromised surface	A						
		B						
		C						
External communicating device	Blood path, indirect	A		X				
		B		X				
		C		X	X	X		
	Tissue/bone/dentin	A						
		B	X					
		C	X		X	X		
	Circulating blood	A						
		B	X	X				
		C	X	X	X	X		
Implant device	Tissue/bone	A						
		B	X					
		C	X		X	X		
	Blood	A	X	X				
		B	X	X				
		C	X	X	X	X		

In many cases, after the biological effect to be tested has been determined using Tables 6.2 and 6.3, specific tests and procedures will still need to be selected. Medical devices come in many forms and the organ that comes into contact with it will differ and it is the manufacturer's responsibility to select appropriate tests. ISO 10993 and its subparts contain procedures for testing but manufacturers may need to look beyond those if they are not applicable. Most test procedures described are based on chemical testing which typically involves extracting any leachable substances from the medical device and using them for dosing followed by checking on its effect on the animal, cells, or other agents. Although this standard provides a recommendation on the type of tests to be performed, additional tests may still be warranted depending on the risk analysis, especially for higher risk medical devices.

6.4 Cytotoxicity, sensitization, and irritation

Cytotoxicity and sensitization are the two basic tests that are applicable to all medical devices that come into contact with the body. Cytotoxicity is an *in vitro* test to determine whether the medical device will cause any cell death due to leaching of toxic substances or from direct contact. Test procedures are found in ISO 10993-5. After it has been determined *in vitro* that the material will not cause cell death, the next step is to check whether the material may cause any allergic reaction to the body due to a potential leachable chemical. This is carried out *in vivo* although an *in vitro* model may first be used to screen the product prior to *in vivo* trials, especially for skin application. The irritation test is the next most widely conducted test and it is directed to the organ that is affected by the medical device. Procedures for sensitization and irritation tests are described in ISO 10993-10.

6.5 Systematic/acute, subacute, subchronic, and chronic toxicity

This test examines the general adverse effect of the use of the medical device over short term and long term usage. Test procedures described in ISO 10993-11 may be used for this study although the main method described is based on dosing a chemical/leachable substance. The standard recognizes multiple routes of exposure and that the most clinically relevant route shall be used. Table 6.4 is the test duration for the systemic toxicity.

6.6 Genotoxicity, carcinogenicity, and reproductive and development toxicity

Genotoxicity and carcinogenicity tests are generally applicable for a medical device that is considered to be in permanent contact with the body. The necessity for reproductive development is dependent on the risk assessment of the medical device. It is

Table 6.4 Test duration for systemic toxicity

Systemic toxicity	Test duration
Acute	Less than 24 h
Subacute	Between 24 h and 28 days
Subchronic	90 days in rodents but not exceeding 10% of the lifespan of other species
Subchronic intravenous	14–28 days
Chronic	6–12 months

generally not required for absorbable medical devices or medical devices with or without leachable substances if there is sufficient evidence to show that there is no risk to reproductive development. All test procedures generally follow that from OECD for testing of chemicals [156–158].

6.7 Implantation

The objective of implantation tests is to investigate the local effects of the medical device at the implantation site. The history and evolution of the tissue response to the implant and the effect of any degradation and integration will be characterized. Tissue response to be determined as part of this test includes:

- Extent of fibrosis and inflammation;
- Tissue degeneration;
- Immune cell response in terms of numbers and distribution;
- Necrosis;
- Tissue alterations such as vascularization, bone formation, fatty infiltration, and granuloma formation;
- Materials parameters, such as any fragmentation and degradation; and
- Quality and quantity of tissue ingrowth.

Analysis of the tissue response may be based on a scoring system where observed reaction is given a score [159].

6.8 Hemocompatibility

For medical devices that come into contact with blood, hemocompatibility of the device needs to be evaluated (e.g., stents, and vascular grafts). The first step is to check whether tests need to be carried out to determine hemocompatibility. Figure 6.3 shows the decision tree for making this determination based on ISO 10993-4. If tests need to be carried out for the medical device, only the parts of the device that come into

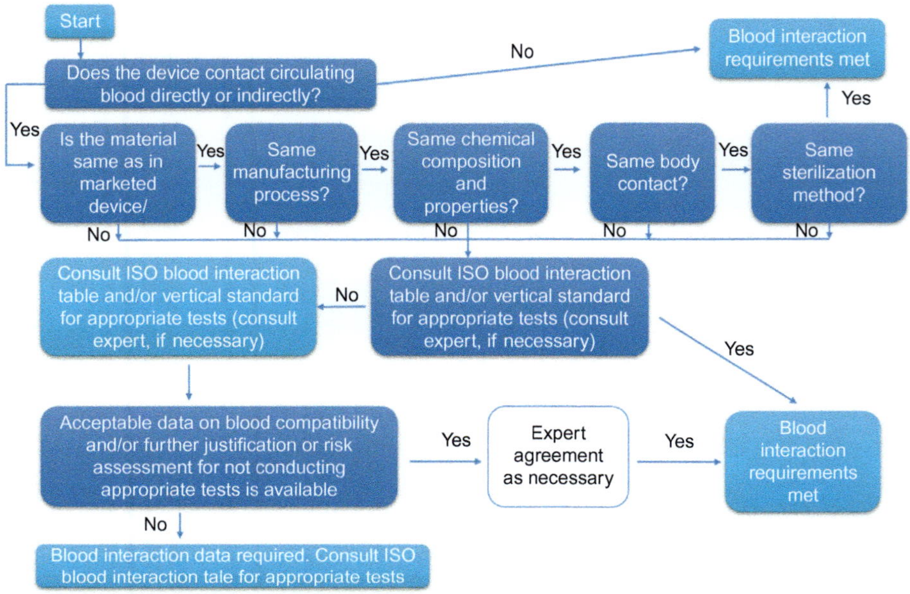

Figure 6.3 Decision tree to determine whether testing for interaction with blood is necessary [160].
Reproduced from ISO 10993-4:2002 with permission from the International Organization for Standardization (ISO). All rights reserved by ISO.

contact with blood need to be tested. The conditions for hemocompatibility testing need to be as close to clinical usage as possible. A device designed to contact the blood *in vitro* and *in vivo* shall be tested accordingly.

Depending on the medical device and its intended use, the method or condition under which it comes into contact with blood may differ. The associate blood interaction hazard will also be different as a result. Examples of hazardous blood interactions are thrombosis, coagulation, hemolysis, leukocyte interaction, and platelet adhesion. A detailed outline of the device examples and corresponding test categories are listed in ISO 10993-4 (Tables 6.5 and 6.6).

6.9 Biodegradation

Biodegradation of a material needs to be considered even though it is not marketed as biodegradable. This is an important consideration for polymer products as they may degrade during fabrication, sterilization, storage, or under environmental influence. In particular, polymer properties can be expected to change when subjected to radiation sterilization. Release of a substance, intentional or otherwise, may come from chemical reactions, leaching, migration, depolymerization, or physical peeling or scaling. Risk analysis needs to be carried out in view of the material and its usage life cycle to determine whether a degradation assessment is necessary. ISO 10993-9 provides a framework for what needs to be tested and documented. It does not provide specific test methodologies on how it is to

Table 6.5 ISO 10993-4:2002

Device examples	Thrombosis	Coagulation	Platelets	Hematology	Complement system
Catheters in place for less than 24 h (e.g., atherectomy devices, guide wires)	X[a]			X[b]	
Blood monitors	X[a]			X[b]	
Blood storage and administration equipment, blood collection devices, extension sets		X	X	X[b]	X[c]
Catheters in place for more than 24 h (e.g., intravascular endoscopes, intravascular ultrasound, laser systems, retrograde coronary perfusion catheters)	X[a]			X[b]	X
Cell savers		X	X	X[b]	
Devices for absorption of specific substances from blood		X	X	X	X
Donor and therapeutic aphaeresis equipment and cell separation systems		X	X	X	X
Extracorporeal membrane oxygenators system	X[a]			X	X
Hemodialysis/hemofiltration equipment					
Percutaneous circulatory support devices					
Leukocyte removal filter		X	X	X[b]	X

[a] As stated in 3.8, thrombosis is an *in vivo* or *ex vivo* phenomenon. It is recognized that coagulation and platelet responses are involved in this process. Therefore, it is up to the manufacturer, to decide if specific testing in the coagulation and platelet test categories are appropriate for their device.
[b] Hemolysis testing only.
[c] Only for aphaeresis equipment and related procedures.

Table 6.6 ISO 10993-4:2002

Device examples	Thrombosis	Coagulation	Platelets	Hematology	Complement system
Annuloplasty rings, mechanical heart valves	X[a]			X[b]	
Intra-aortic balloon pumps	X[a]			X	
Total artificial hearts, ventricular-assist devices	X[a]			X	X
Embolization devices	X[a]			X[b]	
Endovascular grafts	X[a]			X[b]	X
Implantable defibrillators and cardioverters	X[a]			X[b]	
Pacemaker leads	X[a]			X[b]	
Prosthetic (synthetic) vascular grafts and patches, including arteriovenous shunts	X[a]			X[b]	X
Stents	X[a]			X[b]	
Tissue heart valves	X[a]			X[b]	
Tissue vascular grafts and patches, including arteriovenous shunts	X[a]			X[b]	
Vena cava filters	X[a]			X[b]	

[a] As stated in 3.8, thrombosis is an *in vivo* or *ex vivo* phenomenon. It is recognized that coagulation and platelet responses are involved in this process. Therefore, it is up to the manufacturer, to decide if specific testing in the coagulation and platelet test categories are appropriate for their device.

[b] Hemolysis testing only.

be done or recommend any acceptable limits as it is dependent on the material and the product life cycle. Protocol found in ISO 10993-13 may be used to identify and quantify degradation products of polymeric medical devices. Acceptable limits may be determined by other tests such as ISO 10993-5 and ISO 10993-10.

6.10 Sterility tests

Many medical devices, in particular implantable devices, are usually supplied sterile. For a product to be labeled as sterile, verification tests need to be carried out to ensure that the product is able to meet the regulatory body's sterility standard. Traditional and generally accepted sterilization methods are dry heat, EO with devices in a fixed chamber, moist heat or steam, and radiation such as gamma and electron beam. Except EO, other forms of sterilization generally do not leave behind harmful residues. Because EO is known to be toxic, it is a requirement to state the level of EO residue on the medical device following the sterilization process. The FDA uses the following tests and guidance document, ANSI/AAMI/ISO 10993-7, for determining the acceptability of EO residue levels in medical devices. It is recommended that traditional sterilization methods be used instead of alternative methods such as ultraviolet light and chlorine dioxide to reduce the steps for FDA approval [161].

Packaging for the sterile medical device is just as important as its sterility for the obvious reason of maintaining sterility until usage. In most cases, the medical product is packed and sealed in the packaging material prior to sterilization. Radiation sterilization has a distinct advantage in that it can penetrate most packaging material. For other methods of sterilization, it may be necessary to seal the medical product in a primary packaging which is permeable to the sterilization agent. After sterilization, this is then placed in a stronger and more durable secondary packaging material for maintaining the integrity of the sterile packaging during transportation.

For all sterility tests, the test materials shall be supplied sealed in the original packaging meant for market distribution. Determination of sterility is often based on a sterility assurance level (SAL). The FDA requires devices labeled as sterile to have a SAL of 10^{-6} unless it is only intended for intact skin contact; in which case, a SAL of 10^{-3} is recommended. Recognized standards for sterilization are:

ANSI/AAMI/ISO 11135—Medical devices—Validation and routine control of ethylene oxide sterilization
AAMI/CDV 11137 Sterilization of health care products—Radiation
AAMI/ISO Technical Information Report (TIR) 13409 Sterilization of health care products—Radiation sterilization

Devices which come into contact with blood or cerebrospinal fluid need to be verified for absence of pyrogen. The maximum level of acceptable endotoxin unit for these devices is given in Table 6.7. A bacterial endotoxins test or limulus amebocyte lysate test may be used for this verification based on the following standards:

FDA "Guideline on Validation of the Limulus Amebocyte Lysate Test as an End Product Endotoxin Test for Human and Animal Parenteral Drugs, Biological Products, and Medical Devices" (1987)

Table 6.7 **Maximum level of acceptable endotoxin unit (EU)**

Description	Maximum level (EU/ml)
General medical devices (blood contacting)	0.5
General medical devices (cerebrospinal fluid contacting)	0.06

United States Pharmacopeia (USP) <85> Bacterial Endotoxins Test
ANSI/AAMI ST72:2002 Bacterial endotoxins—Test methodologies, routine monitoring, and alternatives to batch testing

6.11 Transportation tests

Care and safety during transportation needs to be determined to ensure that the functionality and integrity of the medical device is not compromised during the process of transportation. Under Medical Device Directive (93/42/EEC) Annex I Essential Requirements, it is stated that the device must be packed in such a way that the characteristics and performance of the medical device will not be adversely affected during transport. Appropriate transportation tests need to be identified and performed to meet this requirement. In particular, the primary packaging for sterile medical devices must not be compromised during transportation. Commonly recognized transport test standards are the ISTA [162] and ASTM D4169 [163].

6.12 Electrical appliances tests

The main reference to the safety of electrical medical devices is IEC60601 "Medical electrical equipment." Most major regulatory bodies recognized that conformance and certification of the medical device to this standard will meet the safety requirements for electrical medical devices. Some of the major considerations for electrical hazards are related to power source, voltage, current leakage, insulation, earthing and grounding, separation of parts, and electromagnetic compatibility (EMC).

Means of protection in the form of means of patient protection (MOPP) and means of operator protection are often mentioned in electrical medical devices. This defines the requirement for reducing the risk of electric shock from the electrical devices and its components. A means of protection may come from insulation having adequate dielectric strength, adequate creepage distance and air clearance, and protective earth connections. Medical devices with parts that comes into contact with the patient or with accessible electrical parts need to have two means of protection. These can be a combination of means of protection listed earlier or by having reinforced insulation or higher creepage distances and air clearances. For example, the minimum creepage distances and air clearances providing MOPP for working voltage of 17 V is 1.7 and 0.8 mm, respectively, for one MOPP. For two MOPP, the creepage distance is 3.4 mm and air clearance is 1.6 mm [152].

Another concern regarding electrical medical devices is risk associated with EMC. The electromagnetic energy emitted by the medical device shall not interfere with its own function or with other devices in the vicinity. A requirement under CE mark is "Devices must be designed and manufactured in such a way as to minimize the risks of creating electromagnetic fields which could impair the operation of other devices or equipment in the usual environment." Satisfying this requirement may be based on compliance with IEC 60601-1-2. However, not all the tests mentioned in IEC 60601-1-2 are necessary. The immunity tests for class I products under CE mark may not be necessary [164] unless interference due to electromagnetic interference will result in an unacceptable risk. There are more than 10 separate tests for determination of EMC, such as radio frequency emission, electrostatic discharge, radiated radio frequency fields, bursts, surges, voltage dips, short interruptions, and voltage variations on power supply input lines.

6.13 Mechanical tests

It is important to consider possible mechanical hazards in the medical devices and to give the device a suitable safety factor unless it is a requirement that it falls within a specific range for its intended use. Mechanical hazards of a medical device may be linked to moving parts, surfaces, corners and edges, instability, vibrations, pressure, and general inadequate mechanical strength for the intended purpose of the parts. Some of the mechanical hazards may be addressed by design without the need for actual performance of any tests. Moving parts hazards are generally caused by the presence of trapping zones where body and limbs may be caught. However, these can be mitigated with proper dimensioning of the parts as given in Table 6.8.

For medical equipment that is not fixed and is not hand-held, its stability needs to be determined to ensure that it does not tip. Such tests typically involve checking its stability when forces are applied on it either in a stationary position or when it moves over or against an obstacle. This also involves checking its movement when it is locked on a ground with a slight inclination [152]. These tests are designed to simulate common hazards encountered during transportation of the medical device.

Depending on the type of medical equipment (hand-held, portable, mobile, fixed), different mechanical strength tests may be applicable to it. Examples of mechanical strength tests include push test, drop test, moulding stress relief, impact test, and rough handling test. Sterile medical devices, in particular those with plastic components, need to be tested for their mechanical strength after the sterilization process. Mechanical properties of most plastics are altered after it is subjected to heat and radiation, which are the most common forms of sterilization. Metals and ceramics are less affected by these traditional sterilization processes. For devices that are designed to provide support for the patient, a safety factor as high as 12 [152] needs to be factored in if the material tensile strength and the external load cannot be determined accurately and if the part is impaired by wear with no mechanical protective mechanism.

Table 6.8 Acceptable gaps

Part of body	Adult gap a mm	Children gap a mm	Illustration
Body	>500	>500	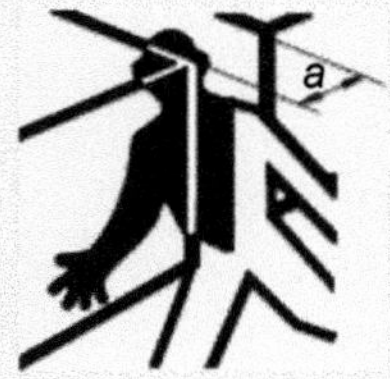
Head	>300 or <120	>300 or <60	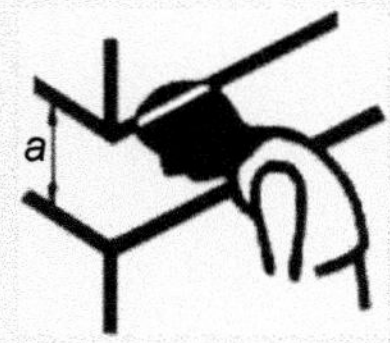
Leg	>180	>180	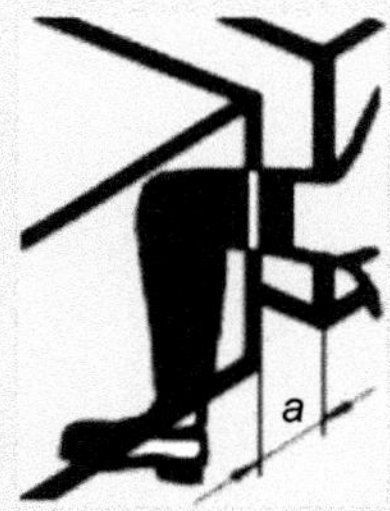
Foot	>120 or <35	>120 or <25	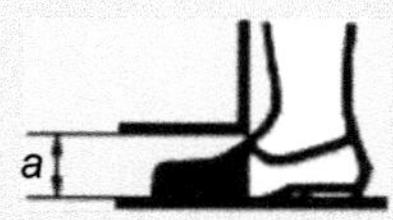
Toes	>50	>50	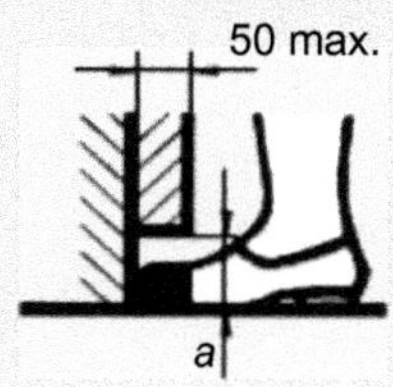
Arm	>120	>120	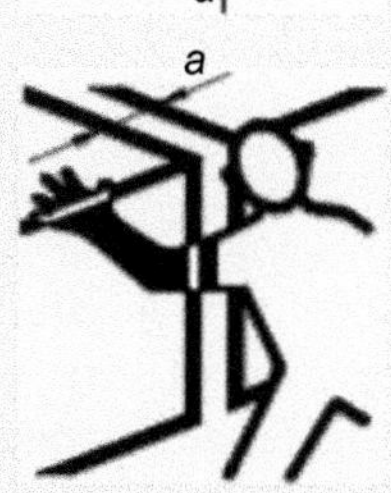

Table 6.8 Continued

Part of body	Adult gap a mm	Children gap a mm	Illustration
Hand, wrist, fist	>100	>100	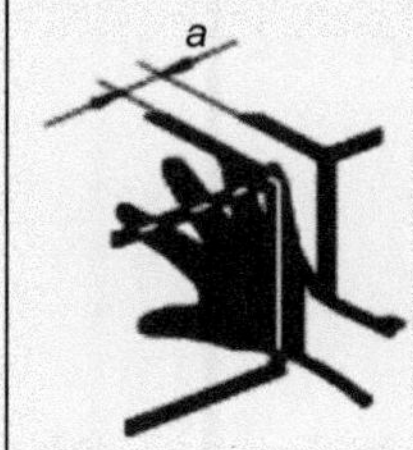
Finger	>25 or <8	>25 or <4	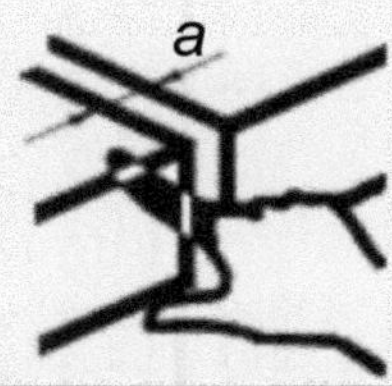

a: The values in this table are taken from ISO 13857:2008.
The author thanks the International Electrotechnical Commission (IEC) for permission to reproduce information from its International Standard IEC 60601-1 ed.3.1 (2012). IEC 60601-1 ed.3.1 "Copyright © 2012 IEC Geneva, Switzerland. www.iec.ch."

6.14 Third-party laboratories testing

Many of the safety tests are outsourced to third party laboratories due to lack of facilities and specialists in-house. The FDA requires the laboratories to be compliant with good laboratory practice (GLP). However, as there is no certification for GLP, the customer may need to conduct an audit of the laboratories claiming to be GLP compliant to verify compliance. An alternative is to look for laboratories that are recognized as GLP compliant by national bodies. Apart from GLP, results from laboratories that are ISO 17025 accredited are also internationally accepted as accurate without the need for conducting an audit as a customer of the service provider. There are also national and international accreditation bodies which certify laboratories conducting tests, calibrations, and measurements according to their standards. Test results from these laboratories are generally acceptable. Table 6.9 shows a list of some laboratory

Table 6.9 List of laboratory accreditation body

Country	Laboratory accreditation body
Singapore	Singapore Accreditation Council (SAC)
USA	National Voluntary Laboratory Accreditation Program (NVLAP) by NIST
	American Association for Laboratory Accreditation
	International Accreditation Service (IAS)
Europe	European cooperation for Accreditation (EA)
China	China National Accreditation Service for Conformity Assessment (CNAS)

accreditation bodies. It is important to check that the laboratory performing the test and calibration services are accredited.

FAQs

(1) What factors affect safety tests?

Safety tests to be performed depend on numerous factors such as the device's intended use, packaging, whether it is sterilized, whether the device is for one time use, and more.

(2) What are some of the safety concerns?

General major safety considerations for medical devices are the absence of toxic substances, biocompatibility, electrical safety, mechanical safety, sterility, storage conditions, and transportation.

(3) Is there an international standard test for determining the concentration level of the toxic substance in a material?

Currently, there are no specific international test standards used specifically for determining the concentration level of the toxic substance in a material. X-ray fluorescence (XRF) is often used for this purpose as it is nondestructive. More accurate techniques such as high performance liquid chromatography (HPLC) or gas chromatography/mass spectrometry (GC/MS) may be used for the detection of chromium and bromine compounds.

(4) How can we determine which tests need to be performed on the medical device?

The tests to be performed depend on how the medical device is intended to be used. ISO 10993 biological evaluations of medical devices, recognized by most major national regulatory bodies including the FDA and CE mark as the standard for selecting the biological tests necessary for assessing the safety of a medical device, can be referred to. To facilitate manufacturers in determining the tests to be performed, ISO 10993-1 has listed the tests to be performed based on the area of contact between the medical device and the patient and its duration of contact.

(5) Which is the ISO for cytotoxicity test? Which is the ISO for sensitization and irritation test? Which is the ISO for systematic/acute, subacute, subchronic, and chronic toxicity test?

ISO 10993-5 covers the *in vitro* cytotoxicity test procedures that are applicable to all medical devices that come into contact with the body.

ISO 10993-10 covers the *in vitro* sensitization and irritation test procedures that are applicable to all medical devices that come into contact with the body.

Procedures for systematic/acute, subacute, subchronic, and chronic toxicity tests are described in ISO 10993-11, although the main method described is based on dosing a chemical/leachable substance.

(6) What are the procedures for genotoxicity, carcinogenicity, and reproductive and development toxicity tests?

All test procedures generally follow that from OECD476, OECD451, OECD421 for testing of chemicals.

(7) Why should implantation tests be done? Which ISO should be referred to for implantation tests?

The objective of implantation tests is to investigate the local effects of the medical device at the site of implantation. ISO 10993-6:2007 can be referred to for more details.

(8) Is the device required to undergo hemocompatibility tests? Which ISO should be referred to for hemocompatibility test?

For medical devices that come into contact with blood, hemocompatibility of only the parts of the device that come into contact with the blood need to be tested. The conditions for hemocompatibility testing needs to be as close to clinical usage as possible. Figure 6.3 shows the decision tree for making this determination based on ISO 10993-4.

(9) What are some of the hazardous blood interactions?

Examples of hazardous blood interactions are thrombosis, coagulation, hemolysis, leukocyte interaction, and platelet adhesion. As such, medical devices that come into contact with blood should undergo a hemocompatibility test.

(10) Which ISO should be referred to for biodegradation tests and documentation?

ISO 10993-9 provides a framework on what needs to be tested and documented. It does not provide specific test methodologies on how it is to be done or recommend any acceptable limits as it is dependent on the material and the product life cycle. Protocol found in ISO 10993-13 may be used to identify and quantify degradation products of polymeric medical devices. Acceptable limits may be determined by other tests such as ISO 10993-5 and ISO 10993-10.

(11) What are the recommended sterility standards?

The FDA requires devices labeled as sterile to have a SAL of 10^{-6} unless it is only intended for intact skin contact, in which case, a SAL of 10^{-3} is recommended. Recognized standards for sterilization are:

ANSI/AAMI/ISO 11135—Medical devices—Validation and routine control of ethylene oxide sterilization

AAMI/CDV 11137 Sterilization of health care products—Radiation

AAMI/ISO Technical Information Report (TIR) 13409 Sterilization of health care products—Radiation sterilization.

(12) What are the recognized transport test standards?

Commonly recognized transport test standards are the ISTA and ASTM D4169.

(13) What are the electrical appliances tests for electrical medical devices?

The main reference to safety of electrical medical devices is IEC60601 "Medical electrical equipment."

(14) What is protective earth connections?

Protective earth connection is a connection to ground or any protective earth terminal for protection from electrical shock.

Clinical testing of a new medical device

7

7.1 Introduction: the role of clinical testing

Clinical testing is the last stage before a medical device is able to apply for registration and enter the market. Clinical testing is a critical step in testing the safety and performance effectiveness of a medical device in clinical conditions. Cell culture and animal studies are conducted prior to clinical testing on human subjects. Differences between a cell culture study (*in vitro*), an animal study (*in vivo*), and clinical testing (human subject) [165] regarding ethics control, conduct, purpose, test object, test condition, time frame, traceability, and study design requirements are listed in Table 7.1. A cell culture study and an animal study should follow the good laboratory practice (GLP) as per Table 7.2 which lists the GLP related area in 21CFR Part 58 [166]. Clinical testing should only be initiated after study on laboratory animals has been done to determine potential toxicity, to confirm its acceptable safety profile, and after the device has been shown to work. Although sometimes the *in vitro* and animal test results are quite promising, it is still not known whether the potential medical treatment that the device offers is truly beneficial to patients until clinical investigation on that treatment is completed. However, a clinical investigation plan (CIP) can be considered at the initial stage of new product development in order to prepare for ethical and good clinical practice (GCP) requirements.

Clinical testing is an integral part of new product discovery and development, and it is also required by the USFDA before a new product can be brought to the US market [167]. EU Directive 2007/47/EC came into force on March 21, 2010 and its Annex X (clinical evaluation) dictates that appropriate clinical data (clinical evaluation) are required for all classes of medical devices, not just those in higher risk categories. And clinical investigations need to be performed for implantable medical devices and all Class III medical devices unless it is duly justified to rely on preexisting clinical data [168]. The clinical pathway usually should be identified at the initial stage of medical device development, followed by a clinical investigation strategy and clinical validation before launching the product. In some cases, postmarket clinical investigations are requested. Clinical data generated from a specifically designed clinical investigation of a medical device are likely to be required, in particular with implantable and Class III devices. Such an investigation must be designed to:

(1) Verify that under normal conditions of use the performance characteristics of the device are those intended by the manufacturer;
(2) Determine any undesirable side effects under normal conditions of use and assess whether these constitute risks when weighed against the intended performance of the device [169].

Medical devices. http://dx.doi.org/10.1016/B978-0-08-100289-6.00007-7

Table 7.1 Differences between cell study, animal study, and clinical testing of medical devices

Parameters	Cell study	Animal study	Clinical testing[a]
Ethics control	Only if cells or stem cells collected from patients, need to get IRB's (Institutional Review Board) approval with informed consent.	Protocol has to be approved before the study by IACUC (Institutional Animal Care and Use Committee). ISO-10993-2 animal welfare requirements.	Application and protocol have to be approved by IRB before the study.
Conduct	GLP (Good laboratory practice)	GLP (Good laboratory practice)	GCP (Good clinical practice) including Informed Consent, Clinical investigational plan and other necessary documents. Subjects should sign the informed consent to confirm the enrolment.
Purpose	Biocompatibility test (ISO 10993), performance effectiveness	Biocompatibility test (ISO 10993), other safety related specific test and performance effectiveness	Clinical safety and performance effectiveness
Test	Raw materials, extract solution, actual medical device	Raw materials, extract solution, actual medical device	Actual medical device
Condition	Clean cell culture room	Specified animal holding facility	Clinical treatment condition
Time and traceability	Short and *in vitro* recording	Short and sacrifice at designed ending point. Record all subjects throughout the study.	Long with follow up; close out at the designed ending point. Some subjects may be untraceable due to patient's personal reasons.
Study design	Statistical difference; different cell resources	Statistical difference; Small animal model to big animal model	Case-study or statistical difference; nonstandardized phases, pilot and pivotal studies, or Phase I, II, and III for 10, 10–50, and >100 patients, respectively.

[a] Partially adapted from Ref. [165].

Table 7.2 CFR reference for GLP [166]

Selected section	Area	Description
Subpart B: .29–.35	Organization and personnel	Qualification, experience, training, sanitation, and health precautions and independency of quality assurance unit from the study unit to assure the integrity of the conduct and results of the study
Subpart C: .45–.51	Facility	Proper design to prevent adverse effect on the study
Subpart D: .61–.63	Equipment	Design, maintenance, calibration
Subpart E: .29–.35	Testing facilities operation	Standard operating procedures, consumables, and animal care
Subpart F: .105–.113	Test and control articles	Characterization and handling of articles
Subpart G: .29–.35	Protocol	Handling of contents, specimen, data, and their changes
Subpart J: .185–.195	Records and reports	Reporting contents, storage, retrieval, and retention of records and specimen
Subpart K: .200–.219	Disqualification of testing facilities	Failure to comply with GLP requirements, communications, actions, and reinstatement

Note: GLP describes the required practices for sponsors to ensure data integrity and quality of animal studies. This table shows examples of GLP requirements.

Unethical clinical studies will definitely shake the public trust. Regulatory authorities should commit to the protection of the participants of clinical testing, as well as ensure that the sponsor (and/or manufacturer) and principal investigator (PI) of the clinical study provides truthful information to those interested in participating.

7.2 Setting up and running clinical tests

Clinical evaluation is the assessment and analysis of clinical data pertaining to a medical device in order to verify the clinical safety and performance of the medical device. Figure 7.1 [170] illustrates the three distinct stages and their flow to the decision tree. The first stage is the identification of clinical data that should include all available published and nonpublished literature and reports, regardless of their findings. The second stage is to appraise individual data sets before moving on to the third and last stage to analyze all the relevant data. MEDDEV.2.7.1 Rev.3 [169] addresses those stages separately in detail. If the manufacturer (sponsor for clinical evaluation) concluded there is insufficient clinical evidence to be able to declare conformity with the essential requirements (ERs) based on evaluator's choice, they should continue to the next step: an actual CIP and budget for another round of clinical testing.

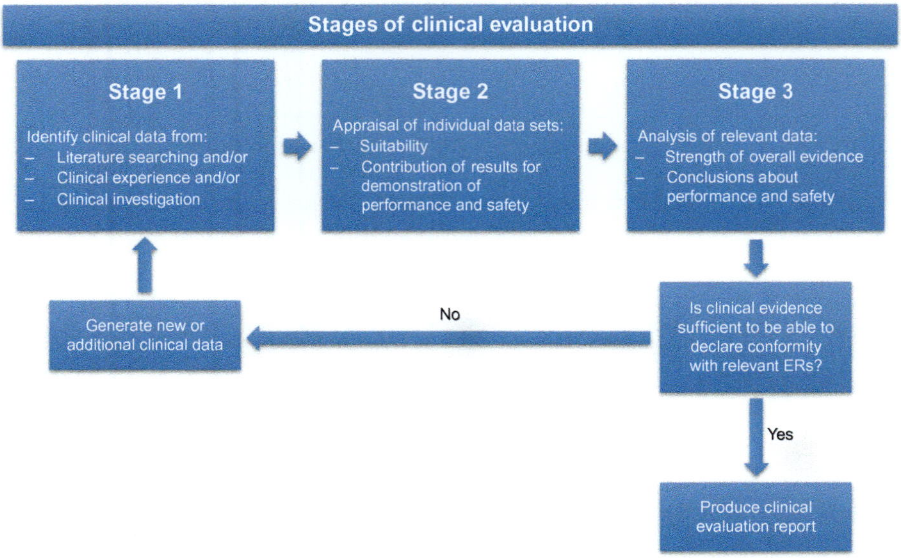

Figure 7.1 Three stages of clinical evaluation [170].

Following necessary regulations and standards related to the specified device on clinical studies, manufacturer starts planning the clinical test: categorizing the device (Class I, II, or III), preparing the budget (by getting senior management's approval), preparing the clinical investigation design, drafting the CIP, and selecting the clinical investigation team and site. In ISO 14155:2011, the CIP states the rationale, objectives, design, and proposed analysis, methodology, monitoring, conduct, and record-keeping of the clinical investigation. It is also a legal document that acts as a contract [168], with the investigation team bound to the CIP (protocols and other requirements), and it also contains the stated clinical testing period and costs involved. Annex A of the standard ISO 14155:2011 provides a detailed format. It should be understood by the investigation team, Ethics Committee (EC) team, notified body (NB) members, and regulatory authority officers. Thus, the CIP should be written in layman's language, with a Flesch Reading Ease Test score of 40–65 [168]. Both the Microsoft Office Outlook and Microsoft Office Word have a "Show readability statistics" option [171], which is convenient for drafting the plan.

The budget for clinical testing is related to clinical trial size (single center or multicenter) varying from 10K to several million. It is also closely related to the investigation sites. Figure 7.2 (cited from Figure 4 in [168], p. 45) shows a relative comparison of budget among different countries using Australia as the base. Japan is the highest cost site, doubling that of Australia. Singapore costs slightly higher than Australia, but lower than the United Kingdom, the United States, and Hong Kong. Other than direct costs, indirect costs such as administrative charges and overhead of each investigation site should be accounted for within the budget; these contribute to about 20–40% of the total direct cost. Typically,

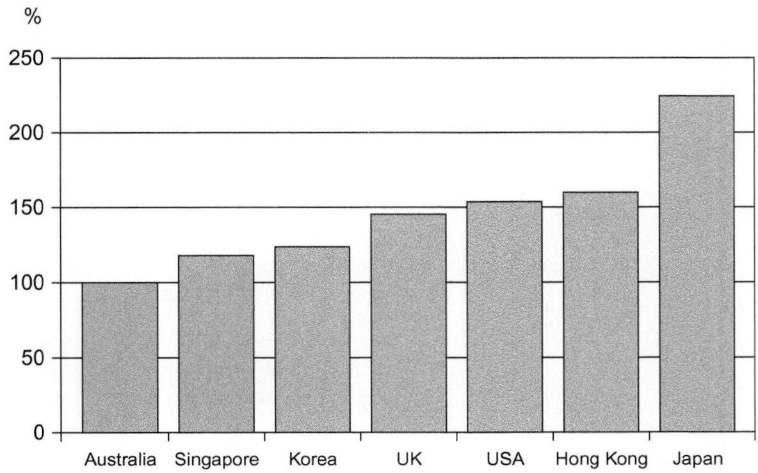

Figure 7.2 Percentage of overall expenditure on medical device clinical investigations using Australia as the base [168].
Permission to reproduce extracts from British Standards is granted by the BSI Standards Limited (BSI). No other use of this material is permitted. British Standards can be obtained in PDF or hard copy formats from the BSI online shop: www.bsigroup.com/Shop.

the clinical testing cost is the highest in the whole chain of developing a medical device: the discovery phase, preclinical studies, clinical testing, regulatory approval, marketing and sales, and postlaunch studies. It is estimated to be over 50% of the total development cost (8 years) for an innovative implant device [172]. In the event that the regulatory authority requests that more clinical trials be conducted, the cost will be dramatically increased. For example, the FDA demanded that advanced tissue sciences involve 350 patients for additional clinical trials; the company continued to invest money at a rate of up to US$3 million per month [173]. Unfortunately, even after the FDA granted the approval in 2001, the company went into bankruptcy in 2002. In addition to the preliminary testing, the regulatory authorities update their regulations and issue new policies for device approval regularly. These new policies might require more tests, including clinical testing. Thus, companies should keep themselves updated on the latest regulations and standards—it is also necessary for them to be aware of changes to these policies. Usually, regulatory authorities will give a manufacturer time for transition and inform them if they do not meet the standard required. Thus, it is very important to keep in contact with regulatory authorities no matter which stage of development the new device is in. Do note that regulatory authorities might have a slightly different conception of a medical device, especially for those combination products. One example from the FDA about reclassification of a Class II device into a drug caused a fivefold increase of project costs and a threefold increase in duration before the product was able to hit the shelves [172]. During the clinical testing, the sponsor and PI should keep each other informed of any information received from the regulatory authority, as well as from the EC.

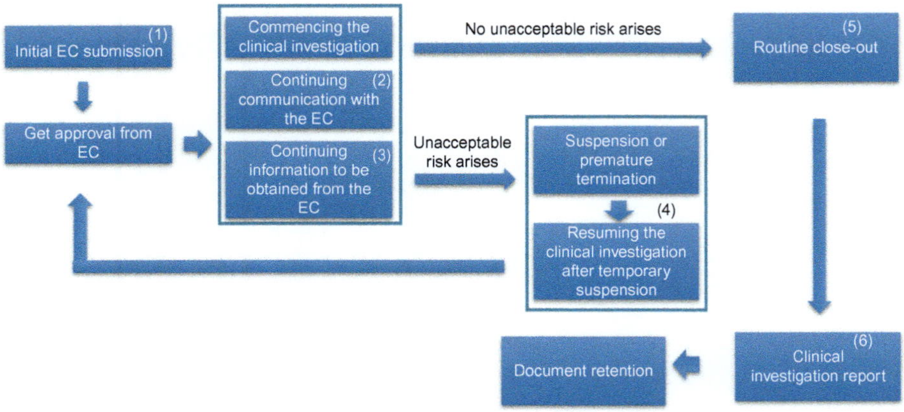

Figure 7.3 The procedures to conduct clinical investigations of medical devices [173]. Reproduced from ISO 14155: 2011 with permission from the International Organization for Standardization (ISO). All rights reserved by ISO.

Figure 7.3 illustrates the procedures for conducting the clinical investigation of medical devices. Getting EC approval marks, the beginning of the clinical testing. A list of documents to be submitted to the EC in Figure 7.3 [173] includes:

(1) CIP;
(2) Investigator's brochure (IB) or equivalent documentation;
(3) Informed consent form and any other written information to be provided to subjects;
(4) Procedures for recruiting subjects and advertising materials, if any; and
(5) A copy of the curriculum vitae (CV) of the PI(s) for which the EC has oversight.

The following documents might also need to be provided to the EC depending on the clinical investigation design and national or regional requirements:

(6) Sample or draft case report forms (CRFs), including other data collection tools, as required by the CIP;
(7) Documents related to payments and compensation available to subjects;
(8) Proposed compensation to the institution or PI;
(9) Documentation related to any conflict of interest, including financial, on the part of an investigator;
(10) Evidence of the clinical investigation insurance.

Reproduced from ISO 14155: 2011 with permission from the International Organization for Standardization (ISO). All rights reserved by ISO.

We would like to highlight that risk evaluation of the medical device must be done prior to conducting a clinical investigation. As illustrated in Figure 7.3, the potential risk should be weighed against the anticipated benefit to the clinical subjects. The anticipated adverse device effects shall also be documented in the CIP. There should be no unacceptable risk arising during the entire procedure of the clinical investigation. Otherwise, it will be suspended or even terminated by the EC (2) (3) (4). There should be written records on all communication content, especially for approval on the amendments/deviations and for notices of suspension and resumption.

Furthermore, the general process for obtaining informed consent should also be documented in the CIP and shall [173]:

(1) Ensure that the PI or his/her authorized representative conducts the informed consent process in the exact way as indicated in the application submitted;
(2) Include all aspects of the clinical investigation that are relevant to the subject's decision to participate throughout the clinical investigation;
(3) Avoid any coercion or undue improper influence on, or inducement of, the subject to participate;
(4) Not waive or appear to waive the subject's legal rights;
(5) Use native, nontechnical language that is understandable to the subject;
(6) Provide ample time for the subject to read and understand the informed consent form and to consider participation in the clinical investigation;
(7) Include personally dated signatures of the subject and the PI or an authorized representative responsible for conducting the informed consent process;
(8) Provide the subject with a copy of the signed and dated informed consent form and any other written information;
(9) Show how informed consent will be obtained and recorded in special circumstances where the subject is unable to provide it him- or herself; and
(10) Ensure important new information is provided to new and existing subjects throughout the clinical investigation.

This process is one of the key points of GCPs, which will be discussed in detail in the following section. In July 2014, the USFDA issued the "Informed Consent Information Sheet, Guidance for IRBs, Clinical Investigators, and Sponsors" draft guidance [174].

7.3 Good clinical practices

Clinical investigations, including clinical testing of medical devices [173], shall be conducted in accordance with the ethical principles that originated from the Declaration of Helsinki [175]. These principles protect the rights, safety, and well-being of human subjects, which are the most important considerations and shall prevail over interests of science and society. These principles must be understood, observed, and applied at every step in the clinical investigation. The foundations for the ethical conduct of clinical research included:

(1) The Nuremberg Code (Year 1947);
(2) The Declaration of Helsinki (by World Medical Association (WMA) 1964, and amended in Year 1975, 1983, 1989, 1996, 2000, 2001, 2004, 2008, 2013);
(3) The Belmont Report (Year 1979);
(4) International Conference on Harmonisation (ICH-GCP) (Year 1995, 1996);
(5) International Standards Organization (ISO 14155 Year 1996, updated in 2003, 2011); and
(6) Code of federal regulations (CFR) 21CFR 50 Protection of Human Subjects (from Year 2012 to Year 2014 annual edition).

In the mid 1970s, the USFDA developed their own set of clinical practices guideline as they found it was necessary to reject the clinical research from other countries which could not reach the ethical and safety standards set [168]. In 1997, the FDA endorsed the GCP Guidelines developed by ICH. On the other hand, the Declaration of Helsinki revision promotes clinical trial registration and results dissemination. In October 2008, the 59th WMA General Assembly amended the Declaration of Helsinki—Ethical Principles for Medical Research Involving Human Subjects. Two newly added principles (paragraphs 19 and 30) considered the prospective registration and the public disclosure of study results to be ethical obligations [175]. In October 2013, the 64th WMA General Assembly further modified these two principles. In particular, paragraph 35 (formerly paragraph 19) requires prospective registration, as follows: "Every research study involving human subjects must be registered in a publicly accessible database before recruitment of the first subject." Paragraph 36 (formerly paragraph 30) promotes the public disclosure of study results as an ethical obligation and states, in part, "Researchers have a duty to make publicly available the results of their research on human subjects and are accountable for the completeness and accuracy of their reports. All parties (i.e., researchers, authors, sponsors, editors, and publishers) should adhere to accepted guidelines for ethical reporting. Negative and inconclusive as well as positive results should be published or otherwise made publicly available" [176].

The main goal of GCP is to protect the rights, safety, and welfare of humans participating in research; other goals of GCP are to assure the quality, reliability, and integrity of data collected and to provide standards and guidelines for the conduct of clinical research. In a nutshell, GCP = Ethics + Risk analysis + Quality Data.

So who should be responsible for GCP compliance? Everyone involved in the clinical testing: Sponsors (Manufacturers), Clinical PIs and Co-Investigator (CPIs, CCIs), Independent Ethics Committees (IECs), Institutional Review Boards (IRBs), Contract Research Organizations (CROs), Research nurses, Clinical Research Coordinators (CRCs), Clinical Research Associates (CRAs), Medical monitors, Data entry personnel, and any other personnel involved all play a part [177].

The ICH GCP is the foundation for developing current guidelines for GCP in various countries. The principles of ICH GCP [178] are listed as follow:

(1) Clinical trials should be conducted in accordance with the ethical principles that have their origin in the declaration of Helsinki, and that are consistent with GCP and the applicable regulatory requirement(s).
(2) Before a trial is initiated, foreseeable risks and inconveniences should be weighed against the anticipated benefit for the individual trial subject and society. A trial should be initiated and continued only if the anticipated benefits justify the risks.
(3) The rights, safety, and well-being of the trial subjects are the most important considerations and should prevail over interests of science and society.
(4) The available nonclinical and clinical information on an investigational product should be adequate to support the proposed clinical trial.
(5) Clinical trials should be scientifically sound and described in a clear, detailed protocol.
(6) A trial should be conducted in compliance with the protocol that has received prior IRB/IEC approval/favorable opinion.
(7) The medical care given to, and medical decisions made on behalf of, subjects should always be the responsibility of a qualified physician or, when appropriate, of a qualified dentist.
(8) Each individual involved in conducting a trial should be qualified by education, training, and experience to perform his or her respective task(s).
(9) Freely given informed consent should be obtained from every subject prior to clinical trial participation.

(10) All clinical trial information should be recorded, handled, and stored in a way that allows its accurate reporting, interpretation, and verification.
(11) The confidentiality of records that could identify subjects should be protected, respecting the privacy and confidentiality rules in accordance with the applicable regulatory requirement(s).
(12) Investigational products should be manufactured, handled, and stored in accordance with applicable good manufacturing practice. They should be used in accordance with the approved protocol.
(13) Systems with procedures that assure the quality of every aspect of the trial should be implemented.

The USFDA governs the clinical trials of investigational medical devices using related regulations (shown in Figure 7.4) to ensure GCP compliance. The USFDAs review of the consent form does not substitute for the responsibility or authority of the IRB to review and approve the consent form and consent process as a condition for the clinical investigation to begin (21 CFR 56.103(a)). IRBs are responsible for ensuring the adequacy of the information in the consent form and may require modification as appropriate (21 CFR 56.109) [174]. The USFDA also endorsed ICH-GCP as well as harmonized ISO 14155 into their regulations.

Recent major changes involving ISO 14155 and Directive 2007/47/EC had a huge impact on the conducting of clinical trials for medical devices. ISO 14155:2011 was derived from a combination of ISO 14155-1:2009 and ISO 14155-2:2009 with several new changes, and it provides very detailed key aspects of clinical study planning, execution, documentation, and better fulfillment of the legal requirements of the Medical Device Directive (MDD) and Active Implantable Medical Device Directive (AIMDD) [168]. ISO 14155:2011 also uses ISO 14971 as a normative reference, thus risk management has to be conducted before clinical investigation. Table 7.3 [173, 179] highlights the differences between the most updated ISO 14155 and ICH-GCP. Both of

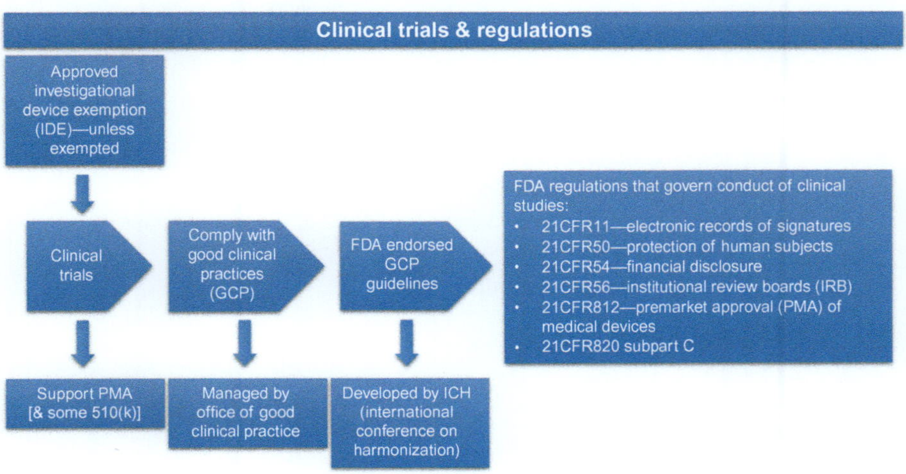

Figure 7.4 Clinical trials and regulations under the USFDA.

Table 7.3 Differences in essential clinical investigation documents between ISO 14155:2011 and ICH-GCP-E6

	ISO 14155:2011 Annex E	ICH-GCP-E6
Prior to clinical investigation	Table E.1	Section 8.2
	E1.2 clinical investigation plan (CIP)	
	E1.7 Log of principal investigator and key members of investigation site team at each site	
	E1.21 Investigation site selection report	
	E1.23 Follow-up letter further to clinical investigation initiation monitoring; correspondence with the investigation site	
	E1.25 Adverse event forms	
	E1.26 Device deficiency forms	
	E1.27 Names/contact information of monitor(s)	
	E1.30 Confirmation of adequacy of the equipment, if relevant to the clinical investigation	
	E1.32 Disclosure of conflicts of interest	
During clinical investigation	Table E.2	Section 8.3
	E2.2 CIP amendments, if any	8.3.9 Certificate(s) of analysis for new batches of investigation products
	E2.12 Updated log of the principal investigator and key members of investigation site team at each site, including signature, title and responsibilities in the clinical investigation	8.3.22 Subject enrolment log
	E2.24 Updated names/contact information of monitor(s)	8.3.25 Record of retained body fluids/tissue samples (if any)
	E2.27 Updates to confirmation of adequacy of equipment, if relevant to the clinical investigation	
	E2.29 Updates of disclosures of conflicts of interest	

Table 7.3 Continued

	ISO 14155:2011 Annex E	ICH-GCP-E6
After clinical investigation	Table E.3	Section 8.4
	E3.6 Notification of clinical investigation close-out to the EC by principal investigators or sponsor, where required	8.4.6 Treatment allocation and decoding documentation
	E3.7 Notification of clinical investigation close-out to the regulatory authorities by principal investigators or sponsor, where required	8.4.7 Final report by investigator/ institution to IRB/IEC where required, and where applicable, to the regulatory authority(ies)
Total document numbers	69	53
Issue time	July 2011	April 1996
Remarks	Specific to medical device	Nonspecific, initiated from pharmaceuticals, applicable to all medicinal products

them aim to make international regulatory approvals easier by providing globally accepted guidelines/standards for the conducting of clinical trials. Table 7.4 summarizes the area of sections in ISO 14155:2011 [173]. In 2012, Giens round table no. 1 was to come up with proposals and recommendations in the clinical evaluation of medical devices [180]; they finally issued eight recommendations to manufacturers, physicians, and policymakers in order to improve clinical evaluation in the medical device field:

(1) Clarify the terminology of certain terms, including clinical evaluation, clinic tests, and performance;
(2) Clinical evaluations must make clear the risk/benefit ratio, the indications, the position in the therapeutic strategy, and the target population;
(3) Clinical tests are not always appropriate;
(4) CE marking data should be more accessible and transparent in a number of fields, including risk management, equivalence, and the drafting of the summary of main characteristics of the device;
(5) Invest in long-term post-market monitoring, in particular in the fields of implantable medical devices;
(6) Raise awareness of medical device evaluation among users;
(7) Extend the interactions between the committee of protection of persons and the world of medical devices;
(8) Adopt and optimize the existing evaluation support programs.

Table 7.4 **ISO 14155:2011 clinical investigation of medical devices for human subjects-GCP (section contents) [173]**

Section	Area	Description
1	Scope	Explains the purpose, principles, general requirements, and applicability of the standard
2	Normative reference	References ISO 14971:2007
3	Terms and definitions	Defines terminology involved in clinical practices
4	Ethical considerations	Describes ethical principles and guidelines for the protection of human subjects of research based on the declaration of Helsinki
5	Clinical investigation planning (CIP)	Describes clinical investigation activities, tasks, and responsibilities
6	Clinical investigation conduct	Describes how the CIP should be carried out
7	Suspension, termination, and close out	Describes the roles, responsibilities, and procedures for the suspension, termination, and close out of a clinical investigation
8	Responsibilities of sponsor	Describes the full responsibilities of the sponsor
9	Responsibilities of principal investigator	Describes the qualifications and responsibilities of the principal investigator

Note: GCP describes the required practices for sponsors to ensure the protection of human subjects. This table shows examples of good clinical practices requirements.

Note: GCP describes the required practices for sponsors to ensure the protection of human subjects. This table shows examples of GCPs requirements.

Herein, we would like to highlight one online registration for clinical trials established by the US National Institutes of Health (NIH): ClinicalTrials.gov [131,181]. Launched in February 2000, this provides a very useful database of publicly and privately supported clinical studies of human participants conducted around the world—until 2014, around half of the clinical trial studies were non-US based. "How to report the basic results" on this online database was described by Tony Tse et al. [182]. Two important deadlines about this reporting should be mentioned:

(1) The Responsible Party (that is, the sponsor or designated PI) for an Applicable Clinical Trial must submit required clinical trial information not later than 21 days after enrollment of the first participant;

(2) Results Deadline: Not later than 30 days after the drug or device is approved, licensed, or cleared by the FDA.

In the United States, the NIH and the FDA have two separate certification requirements to ensure GCP. NIH grantees must certify compliance with FDAAA 801 in their competing applications and noncompeting continuation progress reports for any NIH grant that supports an Applicable Clinical Trial, even if the grantee is not the Responsible Party. An application/submission to the FDA for a drug, biological product, or device must be accompanied by a certification indicating that the requirements of FDAAA 801 have been met. In addition, informed consent for Applicable Clinical Trials subject to the FDA's Protection of Human Subjects regulation (Title 21, Part 50) must include a specific statement about trial registration.

The FDA recommends that a certification accompany the following types of device applications and submissions (including resubmissions) [183]:

(1) PMA (Premarket Approval);
(2) PMA Panel Track Supplement;
(3) Humanitarian Device Exemption; and
(4) 510(k) that refers to, relates to, or includes information on a clinical trial.

This is also applicable to other drug and biologics license applications. The certification requirement went into effect on December 26, 2007. The FDA created a certification form to be used to satisfy the certification requirement: Form 3674 Certification of Compliance [184] as shown in Figure 4.12 in Chapter 4 (with instructions for completion of form 3674 [185]).

Singapore has also established its own online registration system for clinical research: the HSA PRISM online system (http://www.hsa.gov.sg/content/hsa/en/Health_Products_Regulation/Clinical_Trials/Overview.html) for clinical trial application, which was launched and made available to the public through the HSA Web site on September 1, 2012.

It is apparent that, in order to conduct GCP compliance, training is crucial for all personnel involved in the clinical trials. The Collaborative Institutional Training Initiative has a GCP online course for those who conduct FDA regulated research or international research with investigational medical devices and drugs according to ICH guidelines. The Center for Devices and Radiological Health (CDRH) of the USFDA has several related learning videos [177,186,187]. Singapore also has a GCP course, which is available online hosted by the National Healthcare Group [188].

7.4 Reporting findings

Good documentation is part of the ER of GCP. ISO 14155:2011 Annex E provides the checklist of essential clinical investigation documents. Meanwhile, this standard also gives four other useful documents, Annex A–D:

Annex A clinical investigation plan (CIP);
Annex B investigator's brochure (IB);
Annex C case report forms (CRFs); and
Annex D clinical investigation report (CIR).

Based on that documentation, GCP will be able to be practically conducted.

In pivotal clinical studies, professional statistical planning is necessary. According to ISO 14155, statistics are required in the following contents in CIP:

(1) Investigation objectives;
(2) Hypotheses;
(3) Use and selection of controls;
(4) Sample size, and subject size of each center in a multicenter study;
(5) Statistical design, method, and analytical procedure;
(6) Level of significance and power of the clinical investigation;
(7) Clinically relevant endpoints;
(8) Expected drop-out rates;
(9) Performance, risks, and anticipated adverse device effects to be assessed; and
(10) Pass/fail criteria to be applied to the results of the clinical investigation.

The medicines and healthcare products regulatory agency (MHRA) under the Department of Health UK recently launched a guidance regarding statistical considerations of clinical investigations for medical devices [189] in November 2013, which was based on ISO 14155:2011 and ICH-GCP [177]. Meanwhile, the MHRA also launched the "Clinical investigations of medical devices—guidance for manufacturers" [169].

A synopsis of the clinical investigation is a summary or overview of all the key elements of the CIP, such as inclusion/exclusion criteria, number of subjects, duration of the clinical investigation, follow-up, objectives, and endpoints. Table 7.5 gives an example of a synopsis [190] created according to the requirements of Annex A of ISO 14155.

Routine close-out of the clinical investigation, as mentioned in (5) in Figure 7.3, should ensure that [173]:

(1) All essential documents are completed and up-to-date;
(2) All CRFs are completed;
(3) All outstanding queries have been resolved;
(4) The current status of all ongoing adverse events (AEs) is documented;
(5) Arrangements are made for archiving and record retention; and
(6) Documenting disposition of any:
    (i) Investigational devices;
    (ii) Remaining samples (e.g., blood or tissue);
    (iii) Other clinical investigation materials.

Next we move to the clinical investigation report, stage (6) in Figure 7.3. The written form report of a clinical investigation should be completed even if the clinical investigation was terminated prematurely. The Irish Clinical Infrastructure Network provided a good CIR template according to ISO 14155:2011 GCP for medical devices [191]. CIR should be reviewed by all investigators. The archival duties are different based on national regulations. In the EU, applications of nonimplanted medical devices (Class C trials) need to be kept for 10 years, the applications of implanted medical devices need to be kept for 15 years. However, in the United States, the retention period is 2 years after the end of the study or premarket approval application.

Serious adverse event (SAE) reporting for medical devices in the EU is much stricter than other medicinal products. Currently, in the EU, all SAE must be reported within 7 days; this is similar to the Swiss reporting requirement. Each year, the

Table 7.5 Template for synopsis of clinical investigation [190]

Title	
Name of device	*Devl*
Description of procedures	The . . .*Devi*. . .. an investigational device intended to . . . in individuals suffering from . . . The device system is to be used only in accordance with the approved Investigational Plan on subjects who have signed an informed consent form. Device use is limited to the approved study investigators.
Objectives	*The CIP shall identify clearly the hypothesis and objectives, primary and secondary, of the clinical investigation and the populations for which the device is to be used in the investigation. These shall include as appropriate the particular(?):* • *Claims and intended performance of the device that are verified. This may include implicit in the intended purpose of the device as well as those made explicit in labeling, instructions for use or promotional material. It should be clearly stated whether or not the determinations of the long-term effect are part of the objectives of the current clinical investigation.* • *Risk and foreseeable adverse device effects that are be assessed* • *Specific hypotheses to be accepted or rejected by statistical data from the clinical investigation.* For example, Primary objective (may include claims implicit in the intended purpose of the device as well as those made explicit in labeling, instructions for use or promotional materials) • To demonstrate treatment efficacy of . . . long-term dev1 (it should be clearly stated whether or not the determination of long-term effects are part of the objectives of the current clinical investigation) . . . in comparison to . . ., as measured by a . . . For example, Secondary objectives • To assess safety and tolerability of dev1 in patients with . . .
Type of investigation	Prospective, multicenter, randomized, parallel group, double-blind, controlled, etc.
Expected period of enrolment	First patient first visit | Last patient first visit | Last patient last visit
Center(s)/country(ies)	X centers in X country. Centre name, country name
Patients/groups	

Continued

Table 7.5 **Continued**

Title	
Inclusion criteria	
Exclusion criteria	
Comparative device	If applicable
Concomitant medication/ concomitant device	If applicable, please specify (e.g., allowed, not allowed)
Endpoints	
Follow-up	
Statistical methodology	
Study duration	

Adapted from Ref. [190].

USFDA receives several hundred thousand medical device reports (MDRs) of suspected device-associated deaths, serious injuries, and malfunctions. The FDA uses MDRs to monitor device performance, detect potential device-related safety issues, and contribute to benefit-risk assessments of these products. The MAUDE (Manufacturer and User Facility Device Experience) database [192] houses MDRs submitted to the FDA by mandatory reporters (manufacturers, importers, and device user facilities) and voluntary reporters such as health care professionals, patients, and consumers. Clinical investigators must report unanticipated AEs to the sponsor and IRB within 10 working days as regulated by the USFDA, and also report the emergency deviations of CIP within 5 days [187].

7.5 Future trends

An increasing number of countries will oversee and guide the clinical testing for medical devices through a regulatory authority, to protect the patients/health subjects as well as to promote the development of new medical devices. The role of the regulatory authority is to give the approval or objection to clinical investigation applications. Common reasons to reject the applications [193] include:

(1) Suspicion that a device does not satisfy relevant ERs;
(2) Suspicion that the clinical investigation is not subject to controls equivalent to the requirements of the relevant standard (ISO14155);
(3) There exists professional opinion on the proposed clinical investigation which states that the risk benefit analysis given is inaccurate and that, were the investigation to take place, there would be a significant probability of serious illness, injury, or death to the patient or user;
(4) Insufficient information has been submitted to enable a proper assessment of the safety aspects of the proposed clinical investigation to be made;
(5) Insufficient time to assess the application.

Thus, from the manufacturer's and clinical investigator's point of view, compliance to GCP (ISO 14155) requirements is essential to get the approval to start the clinical trials. The good partnerships between academia, industry, and regulatory agencies are necessary to improve the acceptance of GCP for all stakeholders.

Overseas clinical trials are acceptable with comparable healthcare conditions and GCP compliance mainly for reducing the cost and accelerating recruitment. Fifteen global primary trial registries include 205,455 clinical trials conducted in 163 countries from 1999 to 2012, and the 30,964 clinical trials registered globally during 2012 represented a 66% increase from the 18,692 trials registered during 2005 [194]. The largest average annual growth rate from 2005 to 2012 occurred in Asia (30%). Clinical trials are needed in low-income and middle-income countries to address prevalent conditions and improve clinical research training [195]. There are multiple challenges to consider in international clinical trials: (1) complex trial design; (2) regulatory burden; (3) financial and contractual issues; (4) study drug accessibility; (5) quality of data and safety monitoring; (6) personnel training and research education; and (7) other issues like language barriers and time differences [196]. Despite these challenges that can make implementation of such clinical trials difficult, time-consuming, and costly, they are still feasible with sufficient funding, thorough planning, and adequate administrative support [197]. Meanwhile, it is indispensable to the advancement of medical science and the improvement of patient outcomes on a global scale that there be establishment of multinational collaborations among investigators, sponsors, funding agencies, and regulatory agencies. Over the past decade, the Asia-Pacific region has grown to become an important player in global clinical research development and the area has contributed to the provision of quality clinical data to gain market for new products [198]. The Association for the Accreditation of Human Research Protection Programs, Inc., an independent organization, was established in the United States, and even accredited 23 organizations outside the United States, among which there are six in South Korea, six in India, three in Taiwan, two in China, and one each from Singapore and Thailand [199].

Special measures are needed to protect the rights of vulnerable populations, such as pediatric study participants, and shield them from undue risk (Table 7.6) [196]. Pediatric clinical trials should be performed in hospitals that provide a child-friendly atmosphere with a well-defined pediatric infrastructure and supportive personnel to minimize patient distress. While extrapolation of data from adult to adolescents may be possible [197], extrapolation of data from adults to infants or newborns could be very difficult. For example, downsizing devices to fit pediatric patients may change the physical characteristics of the materials used in the device and pose specific risks to the pediatric population. However, given that a device is unique and there is nothing like it on the market, the extrapolation may be problematic and necessary pediatric clinical trials have to be conducted [196].

Medical device clinical trials may require resources that many companies don't have in house, CROs are good alternative options. GCP compliance of the contract CROs is necessary to conduct the clinical testing for medical devices. A CRO can assist medical device companies with clinical trial strategy, protocol design, study management, data management, clinical trial monitoring, biostatical analysis, and

Table 7.6 Protection of pediatric population in clinical studies [196]

Sponsor responsibilities	Description
IRB	The IRB should include members who are knowledgeable in pediatric ethical, clinical, and psychosocial issues
Recruitment	Free from inappropriate inducements either to the parent(s) or legal guardian, or the study participant
Consent	Fully informed consent should be obtained from the legal guardian in accordance with regional laws or regulations
Assent	A child's affirmative agreement to participate in a clinical investigation
Minimizing risk	Every effort should be made to anticipate and reduce known hazards
Minimizing distress	Efforts should be made to ensure participants' experiences are positive and to minimize discomfort and distress

report preparation to ensure that clinical data is collected appropriately to effectively support submission to meet the regulatory requirements. It might be able to realize cost-savings and a faster, more efficient path to market. However, CRO costs are still unaffordable for some research fund scales.

Patients seem to be unaware that by taking part in clinical trials they not only make an important contribution to the advancement of medicine but also gain the opportunity to benefit personally from novel treatment. Sato et al. proposed practical measures for Japan, such as improving patients' awareness and understanding of clinical trials to boost their willingness to participate; the need for this actually also applies to other countries [200]. Implementation of GCP is important to improve the patients' faith in clinical practice, and clear their mind of worries about joining the clinical trials.

FAQs

(1) Is it possible to not conduct a clinical investigation?

Clinical investigations need to be performed for implantable medical devices and all Class III medical devices unless the device is duly justified to rely on preexisting clinical data.

(2) What are the stages of clinical evaluation?

The first stage is the identification of clinical data; that should include all available published and non-published literature and reports, regardless of their findings. The second stage is to appraise individual data sets before moving on to the third and last stage which is to analyze all the relevant data. MEDDEV.2.7.1 Rev.3 addressed those stages separately in detail.

(3) Is there a standard format for a clinical investigation plan (CIP)?

Annex A of the standard ISO 14155:2011 provides a detailed format.

(4) What documents are required to be submitted to the EC in order to conduct clinical investigations of medical devices?

The CIP; investigator's brochure (IB) or equivalent documentation; informed consent form and any other written information to be provided to subjects; procedures for recruiting subjects and advertising materials, if any; a copy of the curriculum vitae (CV) of the principal investigator(s) for which the EC has oversight are all required documents. The following documents might also need to be provided to the EC depending on the clinical investigation design and national or regional requirements: sample or draft CRFs, including other data collection tools, as required by the CIP; documents related to payments and compensation available to subjects; proposed compensation to the institution or principal investigator;

Documentation related to any conflict of interest, including financial, on the part of an investigator; and evidence of the clinical investigation insurance.

(5) Can clinical trials registration be done online?

Yes, in February 2000, the US National Institutes of Health (NIH): ClinicalTrials.gov, launched one online registration for clinical trials.

(6) What datelines for reporting using the online database should we take note of?

The Responsible Party (that is, the sponsor or designated PI) for an Applicable Clinical Trial must submit required clinical trial information not later than 21 days after enrollment of the first participant; Results Deadline: Not later than 30 days after the drug or device is approved, licensed, or cleared by the FDA.

(7) What certification is required to accompany device applications and submissions (including resubmissions)? Where can we get the certification?

The Form 3674 Certification of Compliance that was created by the FDA is required to accompany device applications and submissions (including resubmissions), it can be downloaded from:

http://www.fda.gov/downloads/aboutfda/reportsmanualsforms/forms/ucm048364.pdf with Instructions for completion of form 3674.

(8) What is the online registration system for clinical research in Singapore?

HSA PRISM online system which is available at:

http://www.hsa.gov.sg/content/hsa/en/Health_Products_Regulation/Clinical_Trials/Overview.html

(9) Are there any Good Clinical Practice Course in Singapore?

Good Clinical Practice Course in Singapore is available at:

https://www.research.nhg.com.sg/wps/wcm/connect/romp/nhgromp/trainingeducation/coursecategories/singapore+guideline+for+good+clinical+practice+course.

(10) What are the essential documents of clinical investigation?

Refer to ISO 14155:2011 Annex E which provides the checklist of essential clinical investigation documents.

(11) What are the common reasons to reject clinical investigation applications?

Device does not satisfy relevant essential requirements; clinical investigation is not subjected to controls of the relevant standard (ISO14155); insufficient or inaccurate information submitted for a proper assessment of the safety aspects of the proposed clinical investigation to be made, and insufficient time to assess the application.

Part Three

Practices

Product development overview 8

8.1 Introduction

The basic requirement for a quality management system in product development is the demonstration of project control through systematic planning, review, and documentation during product development. Most of the processes mentioned in the quality management system are already being used in one form or another during product development. Many of the documentation requirements for product development are based on the basic project management process as shown in Figure 8.1.

Proper implementation and execution of the quality management systems in product development will facilitate management monitoring and control of the project progress. The main challenge faced by manufacturers is the demonstration of process control through proper documentation. On the surface, documentation may be seen as non-value-added paperwork that takes precious time off the "real" development work. This results in documents that are missing or lacking in details. Contrary to this belief, proper documentation allows tracking and control of the project and product development without the need for frequent meetings. Scope, resources, and timeline for the project will also be clear for all team members and functional groups while retaining flexibility. Different methodologies may be used in each of the stages of the project management process depending on the company's size, culture, and resources. The quality management system, such as ISO 13485 on product realization (clause 7), requires documentary evidence that generally follows the project management process.

In this chapter, we will use the typical project management process as a guide and link it to the product development requirement in a quality management system. We will also give some examples of documentation that can be used for project monitoring which demonstrates compliance with the quality management system. Most documents are meant to be "live" and constantly updated and modified as the project progresses.

8.2 Initiation

As with any project, there will be a trigger that initiates the process. This could be in the form of customer feedback, sales feedback, marketing feedback, or business strategy. The trigger may initiate further evaluation of the requirements, determining market or customer needs, regulatory constraints, resource constraints, and other factors to determine its feasibility. In some organizations, especially smaller enterprises, this evaluation process may be carried out in informal meetings. However, a record of this evaluation is needed to provide evidence that this process has been carried out.

Medical devices. http://dx.doi.org/10.1016/B978-0-08-100289-6.00008-9

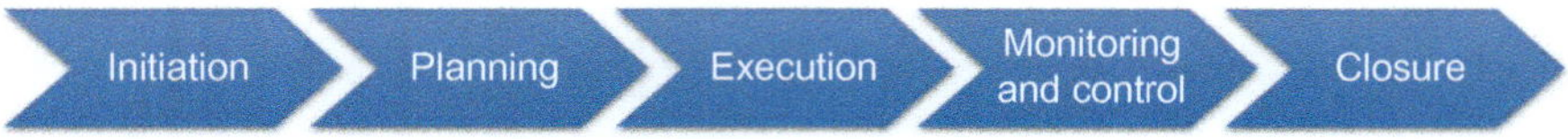

Figure 8.1 Typical project management process.

ISO 13485 clause 7.2 provides a list of minimum requirements for discussion during the evaluation process. Examples of these include requirements from customers, organization, and regulatory bodies; determination of organization's ability to meet requirements; decisions, and any follow up actions. Meeting minutes may be used as documentary evidence that this process has been performed. At this stage, the project may be initiated, rejected, or shelved. If the decision is to initiate the project, the next stage is developing a plan for it.

8.3 Planning

Proper planning is essential for the success of any project. Planning at this stage not only includes the product development plan, but also includes the risk management plan, which is a requirement for a medical device. A proper plan serves as a point of reference for the project team members to understand the scope of the project, clarification of roles and responsibilities, relations between various departments, methodology or process flow chart used, and it highlights important check points or milestones in the development stages. This will reduce project delays, avoid cost overruns, scope and design creep, and failure to meet requirements. Where the project objective or requirements are not properly defined and agreed upon, regular changes and additions to the product will certainly result in cost overruns and project delays. Review of the product development at scheduled project check points as stated in the project plan enables management to keep track of product development and progress toward specified requirements listed in the design requirements document or design input document.

Roles and responsibilities in the project plan are usually defined for the management representatives and the individual departments based on the organization chart. Some organizations may have a separate project department that is fully responsible for the project with members from the other departments (quality department, mechanical design department, electrical design department, manufacturing department) assigned to the project while other organizations may not have a specific project department. In general, the role of the management representative is to ensure availability of resources, infrastructure, and adherence to the quality management system. Roles and responsibilities of the individual departments usually relate to the execution of the project.

Interactions between the various departments and the project development stages depend on the product development methodology which the organization uses. An example of a product development methodology is the Waterfall Methodology shown Figure 8.2.

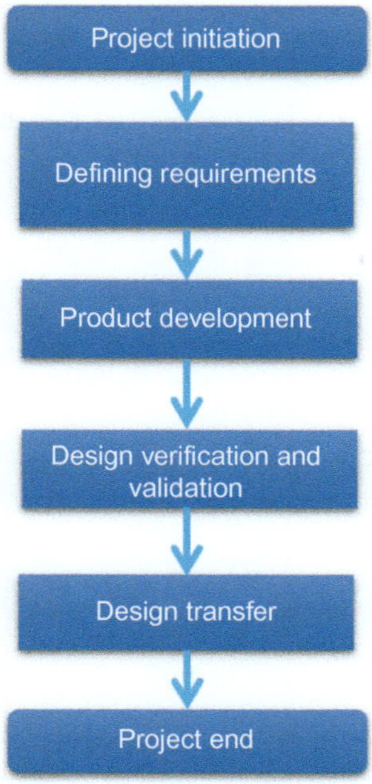

Figure 8.2 The Waterfall product development methodology.

The department involved in each stage of the product development process may be assigned in the flow chart or in a separate table. Each milestone of the project may coincide with the development stages where a review meeting may be called for. The Waterfall Methodology is probably the most basic form of product development methodology with clearly defined stages carried out in a linear fashion. Although most quality management systems do not specify the product development methodology to be used, there are alternative methodologies which may be used depending on the project scope and resource availability. Shown in Figure 8.3 is a Modified Agile Development Methodology which is developed for software development although the concept may also be used in other product developments. This methodology calls for multiple iteration of the products and feedback from customers at the early stage of the development. This addresses a major weakness in the Waterfall Methodology where there is no further customer feedback until the product is out in the market.

The need for documentation in a quality management system such as ISO 13485 should not restrict the organization from adopting alternative methodology. Compliance with the quality management system depends on how the organization frames the product development process. Having the design verification and validation after iterations and the product requirements and design are finalized does not go against compliance with ISO 13485. In fact, the test protocols written and executed during testing of the prototype may be used at the later stage during the design verification and validation stages with a minor adjustment in terms of sample size and the control in the test sample used. Refinement of the requirements is also allowed in most quality

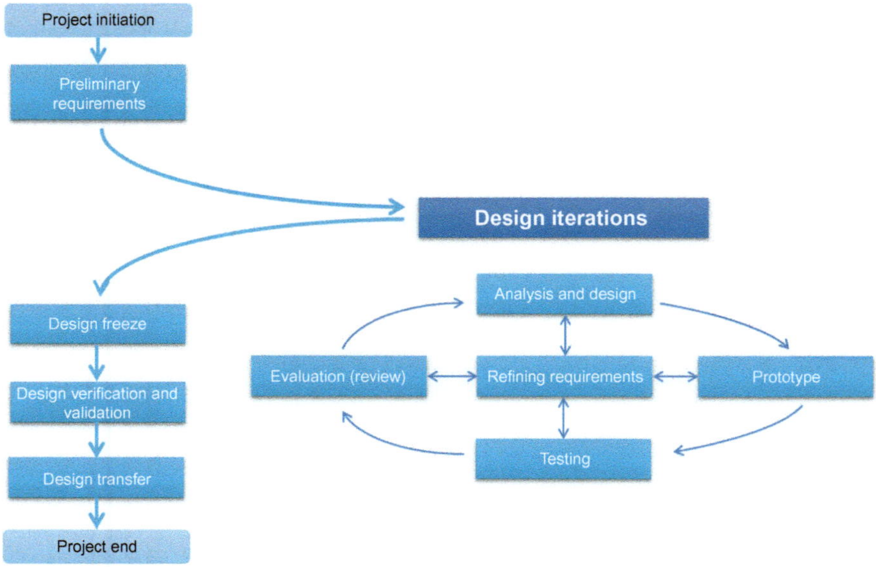

Figure 8.3 Modified Agile Development Methodology.

management systems as long as there is documentary evidence (such as sign-off on the design requirement document and/or meeting minutes) that main stakeholders are agreeable to the amendments to the requirements. Once the development plan is completed, the next phase of the project is to determine the product requirements.

Identification and listing of product requirements is an essential part of the planning stage. Apart from risk-related issues, product design and verification depends on the requirement list to determine whether it has met its objectives. Some of the requirements for consideration include:

(1) Customer requirements;
(2) Functional and performance requirements;
(3) Statutory and regulatory requirements;
(4) Design requirements; and
(5) Organization requirements.

While the project plan sets the high level scope, resource allocation, roles and responsibilities, and the time frame, it is the product requirements which the design team need for execution on their part. A poor design or a design that does not meet the expectation of the customer or management is usually the result of poorly defined requirements. Although the requirements that set the boundaries and expectations of the final product should be as comprehensive as possible, it should not impose too many limitations on the product designers. During the initial stage of the product development, the preliminary requirements for the design may be broad or at a higher level. For example, in the design of a stent, the deployment mechanism need not be specified at the initial stage. This allows the design team to explore various concepts such as using balloons or self-deployment using shape memory materials. During subsequent design evaluations, the management or the team may make a decision on the mechanism and this shall be added to the design requirement document. As this is a controlled document, there will be no ambiguity on the design selection and progress of the project.

There are several ways of determining customers' requirements. Traditional methods include interviews, surveys, and focus group discussions. Other methods, such as ethnography, gather requirements based on observation of the user to understand what they do rather than just what they say. This may involve generation of early prototypes for customer testing and field evaluation to refine customers' requirements. There are a few technologies available for construction of prototypes before investing in expensive production level setups. Rapid prototyping machines are available for plastic, metal, and ceramics. For plastic parts, rubber molding or prototype molding may be used to construct a small volume of parts for testing. This brings us back to the project plan which states the product development process.

Performance and functional requirements are those that may not be specifically mentioned by the customer but may nonetheless be required for the product to meet its intended function or performance. Such requirements are often based on inputs from experts, internal brainstorming, literature research, and comparison with similar products.

To list the statutory and regulatory requirements, it is necessary to first identify the market for the sale of the product. At the initial stages, widely accepted standards such as ISO 13485 for a quality management system and product specific requirements such as IEC 60601 and ISO 10993 may be listed. However, as national statutory board and regulatory bodies are independent of one another, their specific requirements may differ and these will eventually need to be listed. Between EN ISO 13485:2012 and FDA 21 CFR 820.30 in product development, most of the requirements are similar but there are specific differences in the details. In general FDA 21 CFR 820.30 guideline contains more details and emphasis on the product development compared to EN ISO 13485:2012. Some of these differences are discussed in Table 8.1. Further details of the standards and statutory and regulatory requirements should also be included as the project progresses and the other product features and design requirements surface.

Design and organization requirements relate to the esthetic, manufacturing, packaging, cost control, and other business and operational requirements of the product. Cross-functional contributions to the requirements and during the development stage as applicable is therefore important to ensure that there are no unwanted surprises during design transfer and when the product is released in the market.

The risk management plan is slightly different from the product development plan in terms of its objective. While the product development plan provides an overview of the product development, the risk management plan concentrates on the roles and responsibilities of each department in association with the safety of the product. Details of the risk management plan have been outlined in Chapter 5 and will not be covered here. At this stage, a preliminary risk assessment may be carried out to determine the requirements related to the safety of the product. With the requirements document completed, the next stage of product development is the execution of the project plan.

Table 8.1 Differences between EN ISO 13485:2012 and FDA 21 CFR 820.30 in product development

Design Verification
FDA 21 CFR 820 requires much more details than ISO 13485 in terms of design verification documentation. In ISO 13485, design verification requires records of the results of the verification to show that it has met design and development input requirements. Apart from the requirements already stated in ISO 13485 clause 7.3.5, FDA 21 CFR 820 requires the design output document to be verified and signed by designated persons and reviewers. Although not specifically mentioned in ISO 13485 clause 7.3.5, manufacturers typically ensure that the verification tests documents for ISO 13485 are signed off by the test engineer and the reviewer
Design Validation
Similar to design verification, there are more details in the requirements from FDA 21 CFR 820 than ISO 13485. While both require the product to be capable of meeting the requirement for the specified application or intended use, FDA 21 CFR 820 specified that the process consistently meet its predetermined specifications. FDA 21 CFR 820 also requires the validation to be carried out under operating conditions of initial production units. This may be complied by performing the test on production units with their corresponding lot number. It is also stated FDA 21 CFR 820g that the validation tests include identification of the design, method, date and the individual performing the test
Design Transfer
A design transfer document is required under FDA 21 CFR 820 but not mentioned under ISO 13485. The procedure for design transfer should include evidence that there is qualitative assessment of the completeness and adequacy of the production specifications, all documents and articles in the production specifications are review and approved, only approved specifications are used to manufacture the device
Design Change
Design change(s) needs to be reviewed, verified and validated, and approved before implementation for both FDA 21 CFR 820 and ISO 13485. For existing products, ISO 13485 requires an evaluation of the effect of the changes on constituent parts and products. FDA 21 CFR 820 gives more specific requirements such as the need for a master list or index of documents for the product and its production. There is also greater emphasis on the need for procedures for entry, distribution and removal of obsolete documents
Design History File (DHF)
DHF is a compilation of records containing the history of the completed device which includes all documentation such as design plan, input and output documents and validation documents. A DHF is a requirement under FDA 21 CFR 820.3e but there is no specific requirement for a DHF under ISO 13485. However, CE mark does require a Technical File which shared some similarities to the DHF

8.4 Execution, monitoring, and control

A well-written project plan requires good execution to ensure successful completion of the project. This involves commitment from the management and the various departments to the project as outlined in the project plan. Estimation of resources required and schedule in relation to the scope of the project will be tested during the execution stage and it is, therefore, important that the value given is realistic at the beginning. Project team members need to understand and commit to the project plan, their assigned role, and responsibility for proper execution of the project.

Two documents are often used to track the progress of the product development. They are the Gantt chart and the design input–design output (DIDO) document. In project management, a more detailed form of the Gantt chart is the work breakdown structure which typically breaks down the tasks into different levels with specific assignment of duties and monitoring of progress as shown in Table 8.2. However, a simple Gantt chart is acceptable for tracking progress under most quality management systems. The primary function of the DIDO document is to verify that the design output corresponds to the design input as shown in Table 8.3. The input to the document comprises of items from various sources such as design requirements, risk assessment, technical specifications, and regulatory requirements. It usually contains

Table 8.2 A Gantt chart sample

Item no.	Description	Schedule	Responsible person	% Completion
1	Design and development of drug eluting stent			
1.1	Literature Review	02 Jan XXXX to 04 Feb XXXX	Andrew	10
1.2	Listing Requirements	05 Feb XXXX to 04 April XXXX	Andrew	0

Table 8.3 Design input–design output (DIDO) document sample

Item no.	Design input	Engineering specification	Design output
1.	Mechanical		
1.1	A catheter must be able to withstand repeated flexing	Catheter should be formed into a 50-mm diameter coil and straightened out for a total of fifty times with no evidence of cracking or deformity.	<Document Name> <Date and signature of individual(s) approving the output.

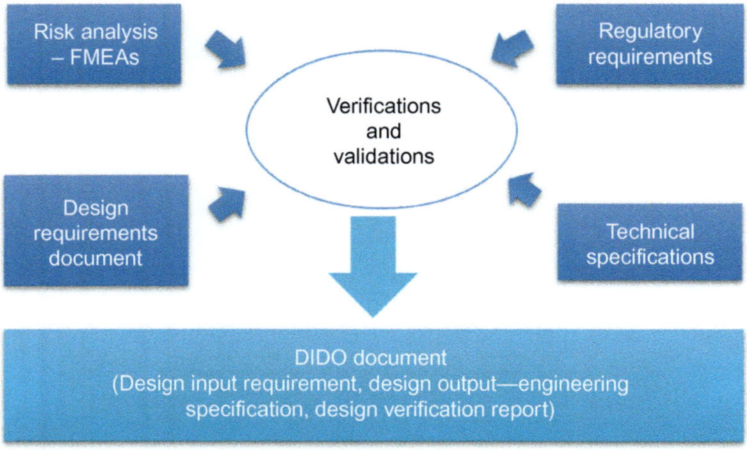

Figure 8.4 Traceability and information flow for verification and validation tests.

all of the requirements stated in the design requirement document and more. This document is normally used as the reference to verification and validation activities. In general, all verification and validation activities shall be traceable to design requirements, DIDO documents, and/or risk assessment as illustrated in Figure 8.4.

In some organizations, the DIDO document is used to monitor the project progress in place of the Gantt chart. This is done by having the output corresponding to the input dated and signed off in the document, which is a requirement for design output under FDA 21 CFR 820.30d. EN ISO 13485:2012 clause 7.3.1 states that "Planning output shall be documented, and updated as appropriate, as the design and development progresses." Thus, it is not mandatory to use a Gantt chart for the purpose of monitoring development progress.

Once the list of design inputs is completed, it is recommended that the corresponding engineering specifications should be added where applicable. This will provide the acceptance criteria during verification and validation tests to determine whether the product has met the input. Customer requirements, in particular, though are often arbitrary. An example of such a requirement might be: the "movement of the monitor attached to the device arms need to be smooth" but it is listed without specific values or a data range—it is impossible to verify whether the product has met that requirement. There are a few ways of getting the engineering specifications. The most accurate way to get this data is by actual testing from internal staffs or customers. An alternative way is to use a competitor's product or products with similar features as a benchmark. A literature search may also yield guidelines or studies which recommend a specification for a similar purpose.

8.5 Verification and validation

Verification and validation are needed to demonstrate sufficient knowledge and information of the medical device to prove that its safety and performance meet its intended use. Contrary to many beliefs, verification is not restricted to performance of tests. Verification activities may be in the form of calculations, comparison with similar products, inspections, and document reviews (drawings, specifications, reports) [78]. Verification and validation activities are often recorded in the design output column of the DIDO document.

There are some fundamental differences between verification and validation. ISO 13485:2012 defines verification as:

> *Verification shall be performed... to ensure that the design and development outputs have met the design and development input requirements.*

The definition for validation was given as:

> *Design and development validation shall be performed... to ensure that the resulting product is capable of meeting the requirements for the specified application or intended use.*

Verification is usually about meeting preferences and specifications set up by the design team under the design input requirements. Examples of requirements to be met by verification activities are weight of medical device, alarm type, signal type, and material performance. They are usually at the component level up to the fully assembled product. Validation is almost always based on the fully assembled product. Its purpose is to ensure that the product meets its application and intended use. For example, a heart rate monitor needs to be validated by tests to show that it can measure and display heart rate accurately. Verification activities for the same device may be tests to show that the sensor is able to detect heart rate and a separate test for the screen to correctly display the signal based on the input. The FDA requires that validation be carried out on initial production units, lots, or batches. However, this is not a requirement for the CE mark.

Unlike research or experimental tests, verification and validation test results must be measured against a set of acceptance criteria to determine whether the test passes or fails. The acceptance criteria are typically found in the DIDO document under engineering specifications to meet the design requirements. Any measuring instruments used in verification and validation tests should also be calibrated to ensure that the test result is accurate and acceptable.

The use of accepted test standards for verification and validation exercises to facilitate approval from the regulatory bodies is always preferred. Because most verification tests are based on component level materials and simple structure, the procedures for them can be found in international standards from ISO or ASTM. The FDA provides a list of recognized consensus standards on their website [113]. However, if there is no applicable international standard, the next best option would be to use experimental procedures reported in academic publications. Without any relevant references to use, the final option is to design your own experiment for the verification test. This is often the case when the tests are performed on sub-assemblies and final assembly on novel medical devices.

8.6 Review meetings

A review meeting is often pre-planned in the development plan document to signal the end of one stage of the development and the beginning of the next stage. The main purpose of the review meeting is to evaluate product development progress against documented requirements and to highlight any problems and follow up actions. This meeting shall be attended by various functional team members so that any cross-functional issues can be identified and rectified. Some regulatory bodies such as the FDA [201] may also require an individual not directly responsible for the product development stage to be present during the review meeting. ISO 13485 requires that review meetings and the attendance be documented as evidence. Typical milestones in product development include requirements finding, initial prototype, product design freeze, design verification and validation, and design transfer. The FDA requires that the review meeting be used as a confirmation that the project is ready for the next stage of development. Although the standards do not recommend the frequency of review meetings, they are usually carried out quarterly or biannually so that stakeholders and team members can be kept up to date with the development progress. This is also an opportunity to review design requirements and to update the DIDO document.

8.7 Closure

Once the product development phase has been completed, the next phase is to transfer the product design to production. This requires close cooperation between the design team and the manufacturing department. A device master record (DMR) as required by the FDA is a good guidance on the type of information that needs to be generated. Required information is as follows:

(1) Device specifications including drawings, composition, formulation, component specification, and software specification;
(2) Production process specification including equipment specifications, work instructions, and environment;
(3) Quality assurance work instructions including acceptance criteria;
(4) Packaging and labeling specifications and work instructions; and
(5) Installation, maintenance, and servicing procedures and methods.

CE mark requires a technical file to demonstrate compliance with the relevant directive(s). This is in some ways similar to the DMR from the FDA. There is no format prescribed for the technical file although it must contain all the elements listed in the annex and the relevant Essential Requirements in Annex I must be met. The following is an example of a structure that can be used for the technical file:

(1) Introduction
   (a) Brief product description
   (b) Intended use, indication, and contraindications
   (c) Accessories

  - **(d)** Regulatory approvals
  - **(e)** Classification of the device and accessories according to Annex IX of MDD
  - **(f)** Conformity assessment route

(2) Essential Requirements Checklist
(3) Risk Analysis
(4) Product Specifications (Drawings)
(5) Chemical, physical, and biological tests
(6) Clinical Data
(7) Package Qualification and Shelf life
(8) Labels and Instruction for use
(9) Manufacturing
(10) Sterilization
(11) Conclusion
(12) Declaration of Conformity

The division of responsibilities between the departments to generate the required information for the technical file and the DMR is dependent on the organization. However, information related to the product design and specifications will likely come from the design team. Additional information that should be prepared includes the material master list and the approved vendor list. The FDA requires procedures to ensure that the product design is correctly translated into production specifications. A design transfer checklist containing the items to be transferred and may be used as evidence that this is carried out.

Proper and complete records of the product development shall be gathered and filed according to regulatory requirements. The FDA requires a design history file (DHF) which contains the history of the finished product. This contains or references records to show that the product is designed according to plan and has met the stated requirements. This essentially contains all the documents generated through the course of the product development including design plan, DIDO, meeting minutes, verification and validation tests, and design transfer records. There are no specific requirements for CE mark and ISO 13485 for a DHF. However, under ISO 13485, there must be proper documentation to demonstrate compliance with the quality system.

FAQs

(1) Why is it important for proper implementation and execution of the quality management systems in product development?

Proper implementation and execution of the quality management systems in product development will facilitate management monitoring and control of the project progress. Proper documentation allows tracking and control of the project and product development without the need for frequent meetings. Scope, resources, and timeline for the project will also be clear for all team members and functional groups while retaining flexibility. A quality management system such as ISO 13485 on product realization (clause 7) requires documentary evidence that generally follows the project management process.

(2) What are the minimum requirements for discussion during the evaluation process?

ISO 13485 clause 7.2 provides a list of minimum requirements for discussion during the evaluation process. Examples include but are not limited to: requirements from customer, organization, and regulatory bodies; determination of organization's ability to meet requirements; decisions; and any follow up actions. Meeting minutes may be used as documentary evidence that this process has been performed.

(3) What are some product development methodologies that can be used?

The Waterfall product development methodology and the Agile Development Methodology are available for reference in this book. There are also other alternative methodologies available for use, but they should comply with the need for documentation in a quality management system such as ISO 13485.

(4) What are some of the product requirements that should be taken into consideration?

Some of the requirements, apart from risk-related issues, that can be taken into consideration are: Customer requirements, Functional and Performance requirements, Statutory and regulatory requirements, Design requirements, and Organization requirements.

(5) How can we keep track of the developmental progress? What other method is available?

A simple Gantt chart is acceptable for tracking progress under most quality management systems. These documents are normally used as the reference to verification and validation activities.

The primary function of a DIDO document is to verify that the design output corresponds to the design input and it can also be used, but the output corresponding to the input has to be dated and signed off in the document, which is a requirement for design output under FDA 21 CFR 820.30d.

(6) What information is needed by the DMR?

The information required by the DMR includes: device specifications including drawings, composition, formulation, component specification, and software specification; production process specification including equipment specifications, work instructions, and environment; quality assurance work instructions including acceptance criteria; packaging and labeling specifications and work instructions; and installation, maintenance, and servicing procedures and methods.

Case study: successful development and approval of a new medical device

9

9.1 Introduction

In this chapter, through case studies, we will further illustrate how to market a medical device successfully with clearance from the relevant regulatory body, how to anticipate potential problems and difficulties, and will provide a further understanding of the role of the stakeholders including the manufacturer, investigator, and the regulatory agency.

The regulatory agency has a critical role to protect the public health through a compulsory registry system with several enforcement tools, but it also plays a critical role in encouraging the development of novel devices to improve the public healthcare situation. In order to help the manufacturer and other stakeholders understand and easily follow the regulations, the USFDA is a pioneer in making extensive use of guidance documents to inform stakeholders of current agency thinking on a variety of topics, although those guidance documents might contain nonbinding recommendations. Now, regulatory agencies in other countries gradually are issuing their own guidance documents to promote local compliance procedure.

The learning curve took place during the USFDA's approximately 70 year history on medical device oversight. Real case study is important for all stakeholders. In 1994 [202], the FDA CDRH requested the Department of Health and Human Services (DHHS), Office of Inspector General (OIG) to generate reliable data on Investigational Device Exemption (IDE) cases before they considered possible revision on the regulations. For educational purposes, the FDA CDRH embarked on an Innovation Initiative to help accelerate and reduce the cost of development and regulatory evaluation of innovative medical devices in 2011. The Innovation Initiative established a Medical Device Technology Innovation Partnership (MD-TIP) which has developed a National Medical Device Curriculum (NMDC) [203]. The NMDC provides FDA-endorsed core knowledge on how to design, test, and clinically evaluate devices, identify the root causes of adverse events (AE) and device malfunctions, develop iterative device designs, and navigate the regulatory process. They designed a series of fictional case studies based on real-world medical device scenarios, and the curriculum follows a format similar to Harvard Business Review Case Studies, and collaborated with many other universities. Case studies materials were uploaded in June and October 2014 on the NMDC website, which are free and available for anyone to use [204]. The target audience of NMDC are students who have little to no experience in the medical device industry. It is very easy for any beginner to familiarize themselves

Medical devices. http://dx.doi.org/10.1016/B978-0-08-100289-6.00009-0

with regulatory pathways for medical device approval in the United States through study of the NMDC. However, those case studies were derived from the regulatory point of view, which lacks comprehensive considerations from the manufacture and other stakeholders. Real cases are much more complicated. Thus, the USFDA encourages consumers and healthcare professionals to report problems with their devices while they are using them, allowing the USFDA to accumulate information on actual products in the national database and take any action if needed for the real cases [205]. In the following sections, we will briefly describe those NMDC cases and then focus on other real cases which are related to registration, clinical trials, nanotechnologies, and software safety issues.

9.2 The approval process

Herein, we are still using the USFDA as a typical example to review the approval process for a medical device. There are three classes which are based on the degree of control necessary to assure that the various types of devices are safe and effective [206]. Identification of the class is the first step in seeking the approval for the device. Class I—These devices present minimal potential for harm to the user and have a simple design—47% of medical devices fall under this category and 95% of these are exempted from the regulatory process. Class II—43%, are categorized as Class II devices. Class III—These devices usually sustain or support life, are implanted, or present potential risk of illness or injury. This category includes 10% of medical devices.

Exemption: If a device falls into a generic category of exempted Class I devices, a premarket notification (PMN) application and other FDA clearance are not required before marketing the device in the United States. However, the manufacturers are required to register their establishment and list their generic product with the FDA.

For Class II and Class III devices, 510(k) (PMN) and premarket approval (PMA) are two routes to getting clearance from the USFDA. Under 510(k), before a manufacturer can market a medical device in the United States, they must demonstrate to the USFDA's satisfaction that it is substantially equivalent (SE) (as safe and effective) to a device already on the market (as illustrated in Chapter 4). If the USFDA rules the device is "substantially equivalent," then the manufacturer can market the device. Only a small percentage of 510(k)s require clinical data to support a marketing clearance by the USFDA. A primary safeguard in the way the USFDA regulates medical devices is the requirement that manufacturers must submit to the USFDA a PMA application if they wish to market any new products that contain new materials or differ in design from products already on the market. A PMA submission must provide valid scientific evidences collected from human clinical trials showing that the device is safe and effective for its intended use.

How to get clinical evidences for the medical device? IDE approval should be obtained from the USFDA. An IDE allows the investigational device to be used in a clinical study to collect safety and effectiveness data required to support a PMA application and in some rare situations of a 510(k) submission. An IDE limits the distribution of an investigational device only to the sites identified in the IDE application. In addition to USFDA requirements, clinical studies of devices are also monitored by Institutional Review Boards (IRB) located at hospitals or other facilities where the clinical studies are conducted. An IRB is composed of medical experts and lay persons. An IRB's approval of the clinical study must be obtained before submitting to the USFDA. The purpose of an IRB's review is to assure ethical principles are in place for patient selection criteria, and that adequate informed consent information exists to identify the risks to patients. The IRB acts as the FDA's proxy to oversee the protection of human subjects who participate in the clinical studies. The initial risk determination of a clinical study (and/or device) is made by an IRB in most cases. The IRB determines if a device/clinical study is a significant risk or nonsignificant risk. The USFDA can overrule any risk determination made by an IRB. If the IRB determines that a device poses significant risk, the applicant must submit an IDE application to the USFDA. The USFDA must approve the application prior to the applicant enrolling patients in the clinical study. If the IRB determines that the device is nonsignificant risk the applicant can enroll patients without submitting an IDE application to the FDA. The clinical study will be constantly monitored by the IRB under the IDE regulations [206].

Cases 1 through 4 in the NMDC in Table 9.1 [204] cover the above general process and most related key topics on how to get approval from the USFDA on a device before marketing. Case 1 introduces the basic concept for the rest of the cases, which provided concepts of classification, 510(k), PMA, fee, and database. Case 2 introduces medical device-related ISO standard 14971, which emphasizes the safety assurance and risk management framework. In order to obtain a PMA, an IDE was introduced and quality system regulations, like GMP, GLP, GCP, were involved in Case 3. Case 4 provides a good practical handling protocol on an SE for a 510(k) application. In addition, a humanitarian device exemption (HDE) in case 5 has been illustrated [196] to show that rare diseases had been included in the consideration of medical device development (Table 9.1). If the marketing area is outside the United States, the manufacturer should seek local regulatory requirements which have been listed in Chapter 2, to check whether they would accept the USFDA clearance or if they require additional routes.

9.3 Lessons learned

9.3.1 Clinical investigation for medical devices

Industry examples regarding the clinical investigation from some real-life case scenarios are summarized in Table 9.2 [168]. They mainly fall into three categories: Need for clinical investigation; Notifications related; and Monitoring related. National differences in gaining medical device investigations in Europe are a major problem for many companies, especially for overseas companies (United States, Asia, etc.). Local language is required or expected, as it facilitates communications between the EC and

Table 9.1 Case studies under NMDC established by USFDA [196]

Case no.	Name	Scenario	Covered topics	Time	Remarks
1	Regulatory pathways for medical devices: Choosing the right one	A fledging company works to bring its first product to market	Comparison of 510(k) and PMA submission, estimated time, review user fees; classifying the medical device; medical device databases	3–4 h	Basic on following four cases
2	Freedom from unacceptable risk: Making a case for safety assurance and risk management	An infusion pump company considers risk assessment and mitigation	Safety assurance and risk management; ISO14971; safety case flow; risk management framework	2–4 h	FDA received ~56,000 reports of AE associated with infusion pump
3	Bring an innovative devices to market: Premarket approval (PMA) of medical devices	A stent company seeks to market a novel medical device	IDE and PMA applications; quality system regulation and cGMP; GLP, GCP; decision for animal studies; determining risk prior to IDE application; biocompatibility tests; nonclinical engineering tests; IRB	Three class sessions	Novelty and high risk level
4	An innovative "Me-Too" IDEA: Premarket notification 510(k) medical device submissions	A hip implant company uses regulatory pathways to speed to market	Predicate devices comparison; 510(k) "substantial equivalence" decision process; specific related standards; 510(k) submissions	Three class sessions	Design
5	Regulatory pathways for pediatric medical devices: Making a pediatric medical device via a Humanitarian Device Exemption (HDE)	A start-up company investigates marketing pathways for a unique pediatric device	Defining HDE; the pediatric device consortia grant problem; pediatric subgroup-age range; HDE path comparing with 510(k), *de novo* and PMA; HUD designation application; HDE application; protection of pediatric population in clinical studies	Three sessions	HUD for <4000 individuals in United States per year, children require special attention because of their vulnerabilities and developmental issues

Table 9.2 Industry examples regarding clinical investigation procedure [168]

Category	Case	Description	Lesson
Need for clinical investigation	Device for gastro-esophageal reflux	A US company developed this device. Following bench testing and a few human implants, the company decided to initiate a randomized clinical trails in centers in the United States and EU because no SE proof with any predicate device. After CE marker approval, it initiated 1-year and 2-years follow up studies.	Clinical data was sufficient for CE mark approval. Before and after approval, safety and effectiveness of devices should be continuously monitored.
	Implant for drug-device combination product	A US company wished to get EU mark approval for combination product after implant obtained approval as a drug. Company assumed that a clinical evaluation based on a review of literature would be sufficient. However, a full clinical investigation was called for.	Class III device and combination products should be considered carefully. The function of combination product would be altered from their separate component.
Notifications related	Ensure all agreements are in place	A US company set up a multicenter trial in five EU countries. No CA approval needed for most centers, however, one center needs to get CA approval before study within 60 days.	DO NOT assume that all EU sites have similar requirement; local requirements have to be met.
	Maintaining an evidence trail	The 60-day CA approval period can also be misleading, within 60 days or stalled for another 60 days.	Importance of gaining evidence of document delivery and continuing to check on the decision process.
	Procedure approval	Ethic committee disagree on some particular procedures, required to amend and seek opinions from radiology experts.	Any procedures listed in CIP will require ethics committee (or call IRB) approval.

Continued

Table 9.2 **Continued**

Category	Case	Description	Lesson
	National difference	A foreign company did not know that United Kingdom has a central booking service to direct company to the nearest ethics committee. France delineated the date protection issued under the national consultative committee.	Check local requirement carefully.
Monitoring related	Standard operating procedures (SOP)	A nurse did not follow the wound care protocol and applied a topic antimicrobial gel, which negated the results for all subjects at that site.	Importance of training and monitoring.
	Sampling	At the interim visit, a monitor selected the same patients and then missed the patient implanted with the wrong device.	Differential sampling at each visit and should match to source date.
	Adverse events (AE)	AD in patient's note, not on the CRF.	No matter AE frequent occurrences or not, should record on the CRF.

their national competent authority (CA). Labeling of the investigation device should be done on the package and IFU (instruction for use), and is required by various local regulations to be in different languages. Informed consent forms should also be prepared in different languages for local investigation site, thus patients will be able to understand the content in their mother tongue. However, it should be noted that any materials in different languages, which are used to advertise the clinical investigation to potential subjects should be approved by the EC before use.

Regarding handling difficulty, a multicenter trial is more difficult than a single center trial. However, in order to save time and costs and get enough subjects within the defined time frame, it is the preferred option of manufacturers. Before GCP was compulsory for IDE clinical trials, audits of four multicenter trial cases in 1995 found several significant problems regarding device tracking, IRB oversight, and informed consent, as indicated in Table 9.3 [202]. The general environment of the healthcare industry promotes the distribution and use of unapproved medical devices beyond clinical protocol design. Hospitals experience pressure to acquire the latest in equipment to compete with other hospitals. Physicians also want to stay competitive as well

Table 9.3 Four case studies on IDE's multicenter clinical trials selected from year 1986 to 1995[a]

	Device A	Device B	Device C	Device D
Description	A prosthetic device with a chemical coating to promote bone growth.	An orthopedic device with promotes the growth of bone mass between two bones.	An ophthalmic device used in eye surgeries.	A device used to treat urinary obstructions.
Problem 1: Device tracking	√ Excess of the devices than approved protocol.	√ Lack of accountability, no record both from hospital and clinical investigator.	√ Lack of accountability, up to 100 extra devices.	
Problem 2: IRB oversight	√ IRB approved limit of 50–75 implants, which hospital records indicated far exceeded that limit.	√ IRB did not follow up the changes of informed consent document; an investigator did not inform of IRB on his movement to other city, 3 out of 10 IRBs determined the study as nonsignificant risk.	√	√ The device number reported by clinical investigator to IRB is different with manufacture record.
Problem 3: Informed consent		√ Obtain informed consent after surgery done; incomplete documents; difficulty reading informed consent documents.	√ Difficulty reading informed consent documents; incomplete documents.	

[a] Summarized from Ref. [202].

as provide their subjects with potentially more effective treatments. Other than this, one possible reason why more subjects are admitted to clinical trials than necessary is that as per IDE regulations, manufacturers (small companies allowed) may recover the cost of developing and testing devices in the investigational stage [202]. The USFDA bioresearch monitoring program (BIMO) inspection during fiscal year 2008 (October 1, 2007–September 30, 2008) identified several deficiencies with regards to monitoring, documentation, and communication while inspecting sponsors, clinical investigators, and IRBs. In 2013, specific to medical devices, common IRB deficiencies are lacking correct SR/NSR (Significant risk/Non-significant risk) determination. Based on the findings of the BIMO inspection, there are a variety of review decisions, and administrative and legal actions available to the USFDA. Major actions are listed here: Untitled letter; Warning letter; Deficiency letter; IRB restrictions on new studies or subjects; Rejection of data; Application Integrity Policy action; Application withdrawal; Disqualification of the clinical investigator; Civil money penalties; Detention/Seizure; Injunction; Criminal prosecution; and Consent agreement/decree [207]. Most of these actions are generally applicable to other violations of the FDCA and regulations, as well as clinical trials.

9.3.2 Nanotechnology-related devices

Nanotechnologists have been involved in regenerative medicine via creation of biomaterials and nanostructures with potential clinical implications. These nanodevices have shown promising results *in vitro*, and some of them have also been successfully tested *in vivo* with animal models. Some successful devices related to skin, bone, cartilage, and nerves are already being tested in clinical trials, as indicated in Table 9.4 [208] and the data produced by some studies are highly encouraging. However, the safety of nanodevices is not yet fully defined and more clinical studies still need to be conducted to translate nanotechnological devices into the clinic applications. Nevertheless, there is still a wide gap between laboratory and medical application of these nanotechnological advances. Meanwhile, nanotechnology poses questions regarding the adequacy and application of regulatory authorities [209–212]. Attention thus far has been on specific occupational health issues associated with engineering nanoparticles. Slower progress has been made on developing adaptations to oversight systems for nanoproducts including medical devices [212].

The Acting Commissioner of the USFDA initiated the Nanotechnology Task Force in 2006 to help assess the previously mentioned questions with respect to regulatory authorities, in light of the current state of the science for nanotechnology. Their report in 2007 offered the initial findings and recommendations to the Commissioner [210]. Recommendations to the regulatory agency included: (1) Evaluate the adequacy of current testing approaches to assess safety, effectiveness, and quality of products that use nanoscale materials; (2) Promote and participate in the development of characterization methods and standards for nanoscale materials; and (3) Promote and participate in the development of models for the behavior of nanoscale particles *in vitro* and *in vivo* [210]. As such, manufacturers would have to make a 510(k) submission if use of a nanoscale material in Class II devices were to qualify as a use of a different fundamental scientific technology. Class III PMA devices are subjected to a preapproval manufacturing inspection and require submission of periodic reports. Any modification to a PMA device and its method of manufacture that could affect safety or effectiveness requires approval by the USFDA through the submission of a PMA supplement. It was recommended that a guide be issued describing when: A sponsor of a Class I or Class II device, who is otherwise exempt from submitting a 510(k),

Table 9.4 Current clinical trials of medical devices nano-products for tissue regeneration [208]

ClinicalTrials.gov identifier	Clinical trial name	Nanotechnology	Tissue	Status/phase
NCTO1539980	Clinical study on Silk Sericin Wound Dressing for Split-thickness Skin Graft Donor Sites Treatment	Device: Sericin scaffold	Skin	Phase 1 Phase 2
NCT01108263	Use of INTEGRA™ Flowable Wound Matrix to Manage Diabetic Foot Ulcers	INTEGRA™ Flowable Matrix (Collagen)	Skin	Phase 4
NCT00317629	Controlled Nitric Oxide-Releasing Patch vs. Meglumine Antimoniate in the Treatment of Cutaneous Leishmaniasis	Electrospinning-controlled nitric oxide releasing patch	Skin	Phase 3
NCT00729716	Comparison of BioCart™|| with Microfracture for Treatment of Cartilage Defects of the Femoral Condyle	BioCart™|| scaffold	Cartilage	Phase 2
NCT01183637	Evaluation of an Acellular Osteochondral Graft for Cartilage Lesions Pilot Trial (EAGLE Pilot)	Bioresorbable scaffold	Bone/cartilage	Phase 2
NCT01218945	Development of Bone Grafts Using Adipose-Derived Stem Cells and Different Scaffolds	Bone scaffold	Bone	Recruiting participants
NCT01435434	Mononucleotide Autologous Stem Cells and Demineralized Bone Matrix in the Treatment of Non-Union/Delayed Fractures	Ignite®ICS injectable scaffold	Bone	Not yet recruiting
NCT00948025	A Comparative Post-Market Study of Commercially Available Peripheral Nerve Gap Repair Options (CHANGE)	Device: Hollow tube nerve conduit, synthetic or biosynthetic	Nerve	Active, not recruiting Phase 4
NCT01573650	Optimization of Peripheral Nerve Reconstruction: A Non-Inferiority Trial	Device: Fibrin Conduit	Nerve	Not yet open for participant recruitment

would need to submit a 510(k) because the presence or amount of nanoscale material would result in the device being outside the scope of the limitations of exemption described in the general provisions of the applicable regulations (see 21CFR §§ 862.9–892.9); A sponsor should submit a new 510(k) for a modification to a previously cleared device that incorporates the use, or increased use, of nanoscale materials; and IRBs, investigators, and industry should seek input from the USFDA on SR/NSR decisions regarding investigational devices containing nanoscale materials. Overall, the report concluded that a new regulatory framework or special regulations for nanotechnology were not necessary at that time, but the agency must keep abreast of the science in order to appropriately apply regulations in the future [210]. Overarching issues for nanobiotechnology oversight includes the role of USFDA regulation, the need for proactive guidance, the adequacy of the current regulatory system, classification problems, and questions of whether nanoproducts are new chemical entities or new medical devices requiring heightened review [209]. On June 24, 2014, the USFDA issued one related guidance document on the use of nanotechnology in regulated products including medical devices [213].

Internationally, there have been similar efforts to spur reporting, though nano-specific regulation is lacking. In 2004, the Royal Society and the Royal Academy of Engineering, commissioned by the British government, recommended consideration of a ban on free (not fixed in a matrix) manufactured nanoparticles in environmental applications [214]. Reports indicate that Canada is poised to be the first country to enact legislation regarding mandatory reporting and monitoring of nanomaterials [215]. The Australian government is considering nano-specific regulation following a 2008 commissioned report by Monash University scholars that concluded that existing regulatory frameworks contain numerous gaps when applied to nanotechnology [216]. In the European Union, in 2005, the European Economic and Social Committee of the European Parliament published an opinion recommending that the European Commission introduce methods to identify nanotechnology risks and propose European guidelines by 2008 [217]. In July 2014, the Scientific Committee on Emerging and Newly Identified Health Risks (SCENIHR) of the European Commission (EC) issued a preliminary opinion on guidance on the determination of potential health effects of nanomaterials used in medical devices [218].

The diversity of nanoproducts may preclude a single approach or framework and instead require different oversight regimes for different product types. In addition, risk assessment for nanomaterials may be difficult. There is little information to date on the effects of nanotechnology, including types and routes of human exposure, dose–response relationships, kinetics and cellular interactions, fate and transport in the environment, and correlations between the properties of materials and their toxicity [212]. Thus, devising appropriate oversight for nanotechnology is a challenge. Table 9.5 lists several nanodevice examples that have been approved by the USFDA under 510(k). It is unlikely to be able to clearly identify the approved medical device nanoproducts through publicly accessible databases of the USFDA as no such disclosure was required for clearance and approval. Thus, there might be many more nanodevices approved than we realize.

Table 9.5 **Approved medical device nano-products by FDA and EU [510(k)]**

Product	Applicant	Classification	Description	Approval date	Remarks
Trade Name: Multiple (NANO COMPOSITE) Common Name: Nano-hybrid Dental Composite 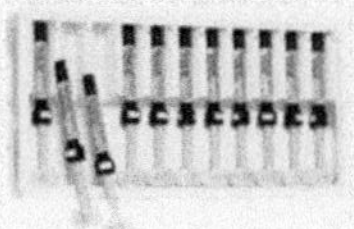	Cosmedent, Inc.	Regulation Class: II Product Code: EBF Classification Name: Tooth shade resin material Medical Specialty: General and Plastic Surgery	Cosmedent NANO COMPOSITE is a light-cure composite resin fabricated from difunctional acrylic monomers and silicaceous fillers. These materials possess physical and mechanical properties that allow them to function in the oral cavity with esthetic qualities that mimic natural tooth appearance.	510(k) Number: K070583 Received Date: l-March-2007 Approved Date: 16-April-2007 Approval Duration: ~1 month	Substantially equivalent to predicate device: Tetric Eco Ceram (K042819).
Trade Name: Multiple (Vitoss Bone Graft Substitute) Common Name: Bone Void Filler	Orthovita, Co. Orthovita, Inc.	Regulation Class: II Product Code: MQV Classification Name: Filler, bone void, calcium compound Medical Specialty: Orthopedic	Vitoss Scaffold is a porous calcium phosphate resorbable bone void filler for the repair of bony defects. It is an osteoconductive porous implant with a trabecular structure that resembles the	510(k) Number: K994337 Received Date: 23-December-1999 Approved Date: 14-December-2000 Approval Duration: ~1 year 510(k) Number:	Substantially equivalent to predicate device: Pro Osteon 500_R Resorbable Bone Void Filler (K980817) Substantially equivalent to

Continued

Table 9.5 Continued

Product	Applicant	Classification	Description	Approval date	Remarks
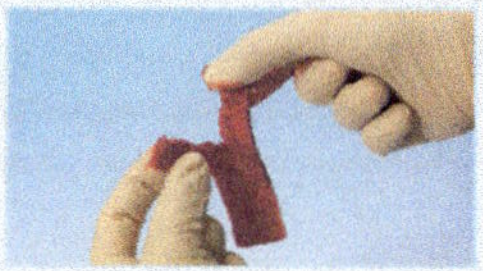			multidirectional interconnected porosity of human cancellous bone. Pore diameters in the scaffold range from 1 to 1000 μm.	K103173 Received Date: 28-December-2010 Approved Date: 7-February-2011 Approval Duration: ~4 months	predicate device: Orthovita's Vitoss Bioactive Foam Pack Bone Graft Substitute (K0S1439, K083033) NovaBone Products, LCC's NovaBone AR(K041613)
Trade Name: EnSeal Vessel Sealing & Hemostasis System Common Name: Electrosurgical open and laparoscopic instruments and accessories Trade Name: ENSEAL® Tissue Sealing Devices Common Name: Electrosurgical Cutting and Coagulation Instruments 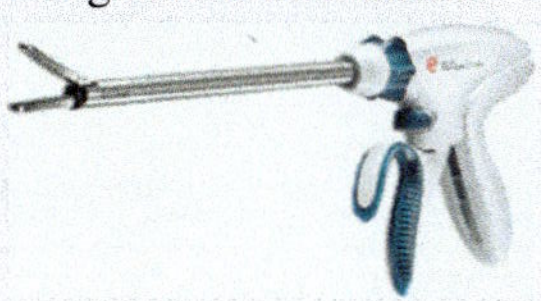	Surgrx, Inc. Ethicon Endo-Surgery, LLC Stryker®	Regulation Class: II Product Code: GEI, HGI Classification Name: Electrosurgical cutting and coagulation device and accessories Medical Specialty: General and Plastic Surgery Regulation Class: II Product Code: GEI Classification Name: Electrosurgical	The EnSeal Laparoscopic devices are tubular instruments with grasping jaws at the distal end, which are actuated by a handle at the proximal end of the device. The Ethicon Endo-Surgery ENSEAL® Tissue Sealers are sterile, biopolar electrosurgical instruments for single patient use. They are	510(k) Number: K031133 Received Date: 9-April-2003 Approved Date: 3-July-2003 Approval Duration: ~3 month 510(k) Number: K13143S Received Date: 20-May-2013 Approved Date: 3-October-2013	Substantially equivalent to predicate device: ValleyLab LigaSure Vessel Sealing System (K981916) Substantially equivalent to predicate device: LigaSure™ Curved Small Jaw (K113572) ENSEAL® Round Tip Tissue Sealing Devices (K072177)

		cutting and coagulation device and accessories Medical Specialty: General and Plastic Surgery	designed to seal and cut vessels, and to cut, grasp and dissect soft tissue during open and laparoscopic surgery.	Approval Duration: ~5 months	ENSEAL® G2 Tissue Sealers (K112033), etc.
Trade Name: TiMesh® System Common Name: Single/ multiple component metallic bone fixation appliances and accessories 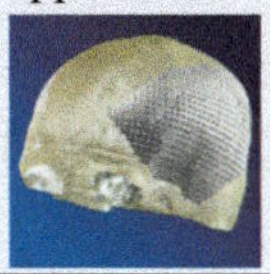	Medtronic Neurosurgery	Regulation Class: II Product Code: HWC, HRS Classification Name: Screw, fixation, bone Medical Specialty: Orthopedic	The device consists of a system of mesh, wire, screws, and plates of various sizes and shapes to be used for rigid or semi-rigid internal fixation.	510(k) Number: K062348 Received Date: 11-August-2006 Approved Date: 8-September-2006 Approval Duration: ~1 month	Substantially equivalent to predicate device: TiMesh® System (K974017, K923419)

9.3.3 Software related devices

The importance of software and embedded systems controlled and managed by software is increasing in the medical device industry, because medical devices are becoming commonly used in the healthcare sector [219]. The use of medical software is an inherent risk to patients, medical personnel, and the surroundings. The intangible nature of software makes it difficult to really know what risks could be present, both user risks and technical risks. A challenge an organization developing medical software faces is to identify a sufficient set of risks for their products. Software-related risk management [220,221] should be included in an initial design plan because software failures in medical devices could potentially lead to catastrophic situations. However, we are still at the initial stage on the risk management of software related devices. Lindholm et al. [221] performed a 2-year case study, from 2010 to 2012, on the software and hardware of a patient monitoring system used to monitor intracranial pressure and calculate the cerebral blood flow. The procedure used in the case study was described in detail in order to learn as much as possible from it, and it has the potential to be used in a medical device development organization or similar organizations. Authors also highlighted the fact that some medical terms were misunderstood by the researchers or the process experts, thus this would be a large problem for the conducted risk analysis. In the risk planning process, the risk analysis should be carried out prior to implementation to avoid unnecessary misunderstandings. Daw et al. suggested the unified modeling language model as a basis for the formal verification of software-based medical devices, such as computed tomography (CT) [222].

A recent revision issued in 2009 to the European Medical Device Directive (MDD) 2007/47/EC made 14 amendments to the original directive (93/42/EEC) and came into force on March 21, 2010. A number of these changes directly affect the development of software for use in healthcare. The most significant change in relation to medical device software development is that stand-alone software is now seen as an active medical device and should be developed following state-of-the-art medical device software development processes. McHugh et al. identified how these changes affect the development company and recommended a specific SPI model to the company in order to conform to the latest regulatory requirements [223]. They are currently developing Medi SPICE to provide guidance for all stages of development of both embedded and stand-alone medical device software. In addition, Medi SPICE will provide a single source for obtaining all medical device regulatory requirements (FDA and EC guidelines, and associated standards, e.g., FDA 21—CFR Part 820, 93/42/EEC, ISO 14971, IEC 60601-1-4, IEC 62304, IEC 80002-1, and ISO 13485). The development of Medi SPICE is ongoing, but it has been piloted in a number of Irish and Australian organizations using a lightweight software process assessment method, Medi SPICE Adept [224,225].

The widespread adoption and use of mobile technologies is opening new and innovative ways to improve health and healthcare delivery. Mobile applications (apps) can help people manage their own health and wellness, promote healthy living, and gain access to useful information when and where they need it. These tools are being adopted almost as quickly as they can be developed. A mobile medical app, like other devices, may be classified as Class I (general controls), Class II (Special controls in addition to general controls), or Class III (premarket approval). The USFDA encourages the development of mobile medical apps that improve healthcare and provide consumers and healthcare professionals with valuable health information [226]. On September 25, 2013, Center for Biologics Evaluation and Research (CBER) under the USFDA issued the "Mobile medical applications-guidance for industry and food and drug administration staff" as the USFDA recognized the extensive variety of actual and potential functions of mobile apps, the rapid pace of the innovation in mobile apps, and the potential benefits and risks to public health represented by these apps [227]. This explains the agency's oversight of mobile medical apps as devices and we focus only on the apps that present a greater risk to patients if they don't work as intended and on apps that cause smartphones or other mobile platforms to impact the functionality or performance of traditional medical devices. For example, a new mobile radiology application gained USFDA 510(k) clearance for viewing images and making medical diagnoses based on CT, magnetic resonance imaging (MRI), and Positron emission tomography on the iphone and ipad [228]. A glucose testing system, monitoring spirometer, electrocardiograph and many other mobile apps have been given 510(k) clearance.

9.4 Future trends

The USFDA promotes the development of novel medical devices by allowing a small business fee. A small business is defined as having gross receipts or sales of no more than $100 million for the most recent tax year. The fee for such a business is much lower than the standard fee [133] or it may even be fully waived for a first-time PMA submission for a small business with gross receipts or sales of no more than $30 million (including the gross receipts or sales of all of their affiliates). As an external factor influencing the innovative actors, the role of USFDA regulation has been unique in the process of open innovation in the medical device industry. USFDA regulations exert a major impact on medical firms' innovation. USFDA regulations govern many activities that medical device companies perform, or activities performed on their behalf to ensure the safety and effectiveness of the medical devices distributed domestically or exported to other countries. USFDA regulations play an important role in the economic success of small innovative firms due to the direct and indirect regulatory costs, especially delays in generating revenues occurring in the commercialization of innovative products stage. In the medical device industry, if product innovation is derived from compliance to the regulations, the innovator needs to involve clinical trials in the innovation process, which could cost millions of dollars, according to William Facteau, Acclarent's CEO [229]. Investigations on how the USFDA's regulations facilitate or hinder innovation in the medical device industry, especially for small firms, are being called for. Because medical devices are regulated by the USFDA, familiarity with USFDA regulations to obtain clearance for product PMA is critical in determining whether the innovative product can be commercialized

[229]. The lesson learned from Acclarent's case is that the success of a medical device start-up depends on how well the company can effectively manage the flow of knowledge to satisfy unmet needs, while integrating their in-depth knowledge of USFDA regulations and third-party payers' reimbursement policies into the product innovation process.

However, based on a survey of 510(k)s that was conducted in 2010–2012, the average review time for small companies is almost twice as long as for large companies and, compared to the EU, regulatory review time in the United States is much longer, thus more US-based companies (especially small companies which are main the innovators for medical devices) sought approval for marketing in the EU first [230,231].

The same survey results also suggest that significant opportunities exist for both the industry and the USFDA to further improve the 510(k) process and the effectiveness of its implementation. Lack of publicly available scientific evidence on the 510(k) process is still the weak point of the USFDA. But, better postmarket data on the safety and effectiveness of medical devices through the USFDA's unique device identification system (UDIS) indicated the importance of the USFDA [232,233]. The UDIS has remarkable potential to improve the data about devices available to physicians and to improve clinical care. Through similar approaches, other regulatory agencies are also able to establish their unique role locally on the development of novel medical devices, while they maintain the safety and effectiveness of devices and enhance the postmarket oversight to protect public health. Thus, more novel devices will be entering the market, and more medical device start-ups will join the medical device industry to contribute to the rapid development of the public healthcare system (Table 9.6).

Public awareness of the AE and risks of medical devices helps to use them safely, this is usually ignored by professionals. AE databases provide original data to researchers who will be able to conduct sound studies statistically to identify the reasons for AEs and propose solutions. Without AE reporting, most probably health regularity authorities will not take action and would assume that current regulations are sufficient. Alternative way of dealing with AEs might be to conduct surveys using questionnaires, but this is not as accurate and may even underestimate the AE

Table 9.6 FY2014 PMA device review user fees from US FDA [133]

Application type	Standard	Small business
Premarket application	250,895	62,724
Premarket report (for a reprocessed single-use device)	250,895	62,724
Panel-track PMA supplement	188,171	47,043
180-day PMA supplement	37,634	9,409
Real-time PMA Supplement	17,563	4391
Premarket notification [510(k)]	5018	2509
30-day notice	4014	2007
513(g) request for classification information	3387	1694
Annual fee for periodic reporting on a Class III device	8781	2195

frequency. For example, Hours et al. established the interference investigation between Active Implanted Medical Devices (AIMD) and Electromagnetic Field Emitting Devices [234] based on a questionnaire given to physicians. Nowadays, we are living in an environment where there are increasing sources of electromagnetic fields (EMFs). EMF sources were basically of two types: electronic security systems (store antitheft gates and airport security gates) and medical electromagnetic radiation devices (electric knives, radiation therapy, MRI scanners), also including new communication technologies (laptops, Wi-Fi, smart phone, tablets, etc.). They found out that the frequency of AIMD incidents associated with EMFs was low (involving only 16% of physicians potentially concerned in France), but nonzero. Cardiologists and urologists were the specialists mainly involved. Severity was relatively low: three-quarters of incidents induced only transient physiological and/or symptomatic disturbance, with minor impact (discomfort or transient symptoms). However, 18% of incidents required treatment; incidents involving insulin pumps, valves, and neurostimulators induced the most severe symptoms [234]. There is increased controversy concerning mobile communication from the general public. Several studies in recent years have analyzed interactions between AIMDs and new communication technologies. Although the numbers of cases are few, they demonstrated that the risk exists and will cause more incidents as the sources multiply and grow closer together. One study [235] focused on cell phone effects inside hospitals, where the need for restrictions is being questioned, and found that, although the incident rate has been reduced by improved electromagnetic compatibility in AIMDs, cases remain in which cell phones impact medical equipment. Occhetta et al. concluded that present implantable cardioverter defibrillator or automated implantable cardioverter defibrillator models seem to be well protected from electromagnetic interference caused by the EU TACS and GSM system, however cell phones disturbed telemetry when located near the program head [236]. Likewise, given the spread of portable music readers, recent studies have examined their impact on AIMDs and on cardiological implants in particular, and found no evidence of interference or effect on implantable automatic defibrillator or pacemaker function. In contrast, Thaker et al., in 2008, reported several cases of interference between iPods and pacemakers, and pointed to a probable risk of interference between multimedia readers and pacemakers [237]. Three approaches to monitoring and preventing AIMD failure were proposed:

(1) Risk-management education by raising awareness and/or instituting mandatory training both for AIMD bearers as a whole and for the health professionals concerned about the issue.
(2) Put forward by patient associations; include training for airport controllers and information posters concerning EMF values to be posted in places such as hospitals, industrial premises, etc.
(3) Encourage AIMD makers to develop even more resistant designs [234].

Of course, we cannot ignore the convenience and other positive effects of mobile communication on healthcare. Lavi et al. described a dedicated cardiac imaging application on a tablet and assessed the accuracy and reproducibility of this novel application for measurement on angiography and echocardiography data sets. They found that this newly developed cardiology iPad application offers the opportunity to accurately present the cardiac procedure in a visual, clear, and professional manner [238]. Understanding of the actual risks of such new mobile apps will help the public to follow the IFU and other safety instructions.

FAQs

(1) Which devices do not need a premarket notification (PMN) application and other FDA clearance before marketing a device in the United States?

If a device falls into a generic category of exempted Class I devices, a premarket notification (PMN) application and other FDA clearance are not required before marketing the device in the United States. However, the manufacturers are required to register their establishment and list their generic product with the FDA.

(2) How can clearance be obtained from the USFDA for Class II and III devices for marketing in the United States?

For Class II and Class III devices, 510(k) (PMN), and PMA are two routes to get clearance from the USFDA.

(3) How does a manufacturer get clinical evidences for a medical device in the United States?

Investigational Device Exemption (IDE) approval should be obtained from the USFDA. An IDE allows the investigational device to be used in a clinical study to collect safety and effectiveness data required to support a PMA application and in some rare situations of a 510(k) submission.

(4) What is the purpose of getting approval from Institutional Review Boards (IRB)?

The purpose of an IRB's review is to assure ethical principles are in place for patient selection criteria, and that adequate informed consent information exists to notify the patients of the risks. The IRB acts as the FDA's surrogate to oversee the protection of human subjects who participate in the clinical studies. If the IRB determines that a device poses significant risk, the applicant must submit an IDE application to the USFDA. Only after getting approval is the applicant allowed to enroll patients in the clinical study.

(5) What are some points to take into consideration when preparing informed consent and advertisement for the clinical investigation to potential subjects in the EU?

Informed consent forms should be prepared in different languages for patients to be able to understand the content in their mother tongue. Any materials in different languages which are used to advertise the clinical investigation to potential subjects should be approved by the EC before use.

(6) Can we check how many nanodevices have been approved?

It is unlikely that the number of approved nanodevices can be identified through a publicly accessible database of the USFDA as no such disclosure was required for clearance and approval.

(7) How are software and mobile medical applications categorized?

Medi SPICE will provide a single source for obtaining all stand-alone medical device software regulatory requirements (FDA and EC guidelines, and associated standards, e.g., FDA 21—CFR Part 820, 93/42/EEC, ISO 14971, IEC 60601-1-4, IEC 62304, IEC 80002-1 and ISO 13485). A mobile medical app, like other devices, may be classified as Class I (general controls), Class II (Special controls in additional to general controls), or Class III (premarket approval).

Global harmonization of medical devices

10

The medical device industry is a heterogeneous, innovative, and dynamic sector. The global market for medical devices is huge, and it will continue showing a significant growth in the future. As we described in Chapters 2 and 4, there are differences between the regulatory systems and required documents for registration in different countries. There are around 60–65 countries which have implemented regulation for medical devices or will soon implement the regulations [239]. The manufacturers must clarify their target markets and comply with the regulations accordingly. For example, a medical device that has been approved by the USFDA may not be able to enter the market in China without the CFDA's approval, even though it has undertaken the most stringent procedures in the world mandated by the USFDA. There is a need for global harmonization of medical devices, and the reasons include:

(1) To minimize regulatory barriers;
(2) To facilitate trade between different countries; and
(3) To reduce the cost of implementing regulations for governments and industry.

But what is medical device harmonization? According to the World Health Organization (WHO), medical device harmonization is a process to encourage convergence in regulatory practices related to ensuring the safety, effectiveness/performance, and quality of medical devices, promoting technological innovation, and facilitating international trade [19]. The European Union is a good example of the harmonization of medical devices, from which the advantages and benefits can be sensed—it was estimated that the European GDP had increased up to 1.5% between 1987 and 1993 due to the promoted completion of a single set of Europe requirements and regulations [240].

Nowadays, different kinds of organizations are contributing to the global or regional harmonization of medical devices, and they will be introduced in this chapter.

10.1 Global Harmonization Task Force and the International Medical Device Regulators Forum

10.1.1 GHTF

The Global Harmonization Task Force (GHTF) was founded in 1993 by the governments and industry representatives of Australia, Canada, Japan, the EU, and the United States. The purpose of the GHTF is to encourage a convergence in standards and regulatory practices related to the safety, performance, and quality of medical devices.

Medical devices. http://dx.doi.org/10.1016/B978-0-08-100289-6.00010-7

The GHTF also promotes technological innovation and facilitates international trade. The primary means by which its goals are accomplished is via the publication and dissemination of harmonized guidance documents for basic regulatory practices.

Most developing countries have inadequate national policies and regulations covering medical devices. WHO collaboration with the GHTF could facilitate access for developing countries (both those importing and those wishing to manufacture) to:

(1) Information on the major regulatory systems for medical devices;
(2) Device approvals and health technology assessment from highly regulated markets;
(3) Adoption of a single medical device nomenclature;
(4) Innovative technology advances; and
(5) A network for postmarket surveillance and vigilance.

The medical devices team at WHO welcomed the chairmanship of the European Union of the GHTF in 2004 and the opportunity to identify areas and mechanisms for increased collaboration, including an observer role on the Steering Committee and Vigilance Study Group.

The GHTF had four study groups [19], and the scope of each group is shown in Figure 10.1.

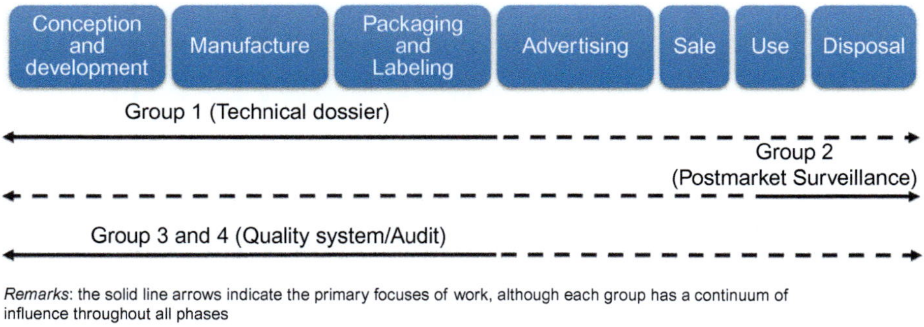

Figure 10.1 Scope of the four GHTF study groups.
Reprinted from Medical device regulations: global overview and guiding principles, WHO, Chapter 2. Medical device safety, 5 pp., Copyright (2003).

10.1.2 IMDRF

The International Medical Device Regulators Forum (IMDRF) was conceived in February 2011 as a forum to discuss future directions in medical device regulatory harmonization [241].

It is a voluntary group of medical device regulators from around the world who have come together to build on the strong foundational work of the Global Harmonization Task Force on Medical Devices (GHTF) and to accelerate international medical device regulatory harmonization and convergence.

The IMDRF was born in October 2011, when representatives from the medical device regulatory authorities of Australia, Brazil, Canada, China, the European Union, Japan, and the United States, as well as the WHO met in Ottawa to address the establishment and operation of this new Forum.

The IMDRF Management Committee comprises regulatory authority representatives from the following jurisdictions:

(1) Australia, Therapeutic Goods Administration;
(2) Brazil, National Health Surveillance Agency (ANVISA);
(3) Canada, Health Canada;
(4) Europe, European Commission Directorate General Health and Consumers;
(5) Japan, Pharmaceuticals and Medical Devices Agency and the Ministry of Health, Labour and Welfare;
(6) Russia, Russian Ministry of Health; and
(7) United States of America, US Food and Drug Administration.

The IMDRF Management Committee meets biannually. The first meeting was held in Singapore February 28 to March 1, 2012 [242].

More information about IMDRF can be found at: http://www.imdrf.org/.

10.2 Working Parties in each continent

10.2.1 Asian Harmonization Working Party

The Asian Harmonization Working Party (AHWP) was established as a nonprofit organization. Its goals are to study and recommend ways to harmonize medical device regulations in the Asian and other regions, to work in coordination with the Global Harmonization Task Force, APEC, and other related international organizations aiming at establishing harmonized requirements, procedures, and standards. The Working Party is a group of experts from the medical device regulatory authorities and the medical device industry. Membership is open to representatives from the Asian and other regions that support the above stated goals [243]. The AHWP contains 24 member economies, and they are:

(1) Abu Dhabi;
(2) Brunei Darussalam;
(3) Cambodia;
(4) Chile;
(5) Chinese Taipei;
(6) Hong Kong SAR, China;
(7) India;
(8) Indonesia;
(9) Jordan;
(10) Kingdom of Saudi Arabia;
(11) Republic of Korea;
(12) Laos;
(13) Malaysia;
(14) Myanmar;
(15) Pakistan;
(16) People's Republic of China;
(17) Philippines;

(18) Singapore;
(19) South Africa;
(20) State of Kuwait;
(21) Tanzania;
(22) Thailand;
(23) Vietnam; and
(24) Yemen.

More information about AHWP can be found at: http://www.ahwp.info/.

10.2.2 Pan American Network for Drug Regulatory Harmonization

The Pan American Network for Drug Regulatory Harmonization (PANDRH) is an initiative of the national regulatory authorities within the Region, and Pan American Health Organization (PAHO), that supports the processes of pharmaceutical regulatory harmonization in the Americas, within the framework of national and subregional health policies and recognizing preexisting asymmetries [244].

The components of PANDRH are: The Pan American Conference on Drug Regulatory Harmonization (PANDHR), the Steering Committee (SC), the Technical Working Groups (WGs) in the areas considered as priority by the Conference and the Secretariat.

There are 13 working groups within PANDRH, and they are:

(1) Bioequivalence;
(2) Biotechnological products;
(3) Counterfeit medicines;
(4) Good Clinical Practices;
(5) Good Laboratory Practices;
(6) Good Manufacturing Practices;
(7) Medical Plants;
(8) Medicines Classification;
(9) Medicines Promotion;
(10) Medicines Registration;
(11) Pharmacopoeia;
(12) Pharmacovigilance; and
(13) Vaccines.

More information about PANDRH can be found at: http://www.paho.org/hq/index.php?option=com_content&view=category&id=1156&layout=blog&Itemid=1685&lang=en.

10.2.3 Pan African Harmonization Working Party on Medical Devices and Diagnostics

The Pan African Harmonization Working Party (PAHWP) is a voluntary body that aims to improve access to safe and affordable medical devices and diagnostics in Africa though harmonized regulation. The first priority is *in vitro* diagnostic devices. A new generation of diagnostic tests are being developed for use at the point of care that could save lives and stop the spread of infectious diseases. It is important that patients in Africa have access to these tests without delay [245].

The PAHWP aims to study and recommend ways to ensure tests are safe and effective while minimizing costs and delays, allowing faster access to cheaper products. The PAHWP undertakes pilot projects in Africa using new point-of-care tests for CD4, viral load, and early infant diagnosis of HIV, as examples.

The PAHWP is housed under the African Union-New Partnership for Africa's Development (AU-NEPAD) Planning and Coordinating Agency. Founding members include the East African Community Health Secretariat (EAC) and the EAC partner states, Ethiopia, Nigeria, and South Africa and the London School of Hygiene & Tropical Medicine. Partners include the German International Co-operation (EAC-GIZ), the African Society for Laboratory Medicine (ASLM), and the World Health Organization (AFRO, WHO). Companies that develop and manufacture IVD Medical Devices are partners and PAHWP is currently expanding through the incorporation of Southern African Development Community (SADC) Partner States.

The project is facilitated by the London School of Hygiene & Tropical Medicine (LSHTM) with grant funding from Grand Challenges Canada (GCC). The PAHWP is collaborating with the AHWP and the Latin America IVD Association (ALADDIV).

More information about PAHWP can be found at: http://www.pahwp.org/.

10.3 Other societies

10.3.1 Regulatory Affairs Professionals Society

The Regulatory Affairs Professionals Society (RAPS) is the largest global organization involved with the regulation of healthcare and related products, including medical devices, pharmaceuticals, biologics, and nutritional products. Founded in 1976, RAPS helped establish the regulatory profession and continues to actively support the professional and lead the profession as a neutral, nonlobbying, nonprofit organization. RAPS offers education and training, professional standards, publications, research, knowledge sharing, networking, career development opportunities and other valuable resources, including Regulatory Affairs Certification (RAC), the only postacademic professional credential to recognize regulatory excellence. RAPS is headquartered in suburban Washington, DC, with offices in Shanghai and Singapore and chapters and affiliates worldwide [246].

Its mission is to create and promote a clear identity for the regulatory professional, establish standards for the profession, assure access to resources to meet the standards, and recognize achievement.

More information about RAPS can be found at: http://www.raps.org/.

10.3.2 ASEAN Alliance of Health Supplement Associations

The ASEAN Alliance of Health Supplement Associations (AAHSA) was created in 2006 to work with the regulatory bodies of ASEAN to achieve harmonization in health supplements across the region by 2015. The AAHSA now brings together seven national health supplement associations which work closely with their national authorities on legislation and collaborate on regional issues.

The AAHSA recognizes that its role in the ASEAN harmonization process is to provide access to its extensive regional and international scientific, technical expertise and to provide guidance on how any regulatory framework being developed will impact the market.

The AAHSA is committed to regional harmonization to help create a "domestic market" with the scale to allow ASEAN companies to compete effectively in the global marketplace, and to make the ASEAN an even more attractive location for companies to place their regional or global manufacturing and research and development facilities.

While the AAHSA recognizes the importance of harmonization and the creation of the ASEAN Economic Community, it is also conscious that any regulatory framework must meet the following three criteria:

(1) It must be suitably clear, practical, and workable to be implemented equally in all countries and applied by companies in the sector, both large and small;
(2) It must rely on the best international science; and
(3) It must reflect the unique characteristics of health supplement products and seek to find specific regulatory solutions that ensure quality and safety without compromising consumer choice.

The AAHSA sees a very bright future for the health supplement sector in the ASEAN with an increasing role in creating healthier communities [247].

More information about AAHSA can be found at: http://www.aahsa.org.sg/.

FAQs

(1) Why is there a need for global harmonization of medical devices?

Global harmonization is needed to minimize regulatory barriers, facilitate trade between different countries, and reduce the cost of implementing regulations for governments and industry.

(2) How are the World Health Organization (WHO) and Global Harmonization Task Force (GHTF) involved in helping developing countries?

WHO collaboration with the GHTF could facilitate access for developing countries to information on the major regulatory systems for medical devices; device approvals and health technology assessment from highly regulated markets; adoption of a single medical device nomenclature; innovative technology advances; and a network for postmarket surveillance and vigilance.

(3) What is the purpose of the Asian Harmonization Working Party (AHWP)?

The goals of the Asian Harmonization Working Party (AHWP) are to study and recommend ways to harmonize medical device regulations in Asia and other regions and to work in coordination with the Global Harmonization Task Force, APEC, and other related international organizations aiming at establishing harmonized requirements, procedures, and standards.

(4) What is the goal of the International Medical Device Regulators Forum (IMDRF) and Global Harmonization Task Force (GHTF)?

IMDRF and GHTP work together to expedite international medical device regulatory harmonization and convergence.

(5) What is the aim of the Pan African Harmonization Working Party on Medical Devices and Diagnostics (PAHWP)?

The PAHWP aims to improve access to safe and affordable medical devices and diagnostics in Africa through harmonized regulation, and to study and recommend ways to ensure tests are safe and effective while minimizing costs and delays, allowing faster access to cheaper products.

(6) What are the functions of the Regulatory Affairs Professionals Society (RAPS)?

RAPS is involved with the regulation of healthcare and related products, including medical devices, pharmaceuticals, biologics, and nutritional products. RAPS helped establish the regulatory profession and continues to actively support the professional and lead the profession as a neutral, nonlobbying, nonprofit organization. RAPS also offers education and training, professional standards, publications, research, knowledge sharing, networking, career development opportunities, and other valuable resources, including Regulatory Affairs Certification (RAC).

(7) What are the criteria for a regulatory framework?

The regulatory framework must be suitably clear, practical, and workable to be implemented equally in all countries and applied by companies in the sector, both large and small. It must rely on the best international science and it must reflect the unique characteristics of health supplement products and seek to find specific regulatory solutions that ensure quality and safety without compromising consumer choice.

References

[1] U.S. Food and Drug Administration, Is the product a medical device? Retrieved December 09, 2014, from http://www.fda.gov/MedicalDevices/DeviceRegulationandGuidance/Overview/ClassifyYourDevice/ucm051512.htm, 2014.

[2] Study Group 1 of the Global Harmonization Task Force, Definition of the Terms 'Medical Device' and 'In Vitro Diagnostic (IVD) Medical Device', from http://www.google.com.sg/url?sa=t&rct=j&q=&esrc=s&source=web&cd=1&cad=rja&uact=8&ved=0CBwQFjAA&url=http%3A%2F%2Fwww.imdrf.org%2Fdocs%2Fghtf%2Ffinal%2Fsg1%2Ftechnical-docs%2Fghtf-sg1-n071-2012-definition-of-terms-120516.docx&ei=M7iOVPO1LMewuASwlYLoBA&usg=AFQjCNEA8bFerfd8m5uyHC4DMHyT6v8afQ&sig2=K9ijNzysaF_SM0XamIdhVQ&bvm=bv.81828268,d.c2E, 2012.

[3] The European Parliment and the Council of the European Union, Directive 2007/47/EC of the European Parliment and of the Council, Official J. Eur. Union 247 (2007) 21–55.

[4] International Organization for Standardization, ISO13485:2012. Medical devices—quality management systems—requirements for regulatory purposes, 2012.

[5] A. Morse, Novartis and Google to work on smart contact lenses. Retrieved October 10, 2014, from http://www.wsj.com/articles/novatis-google-to-work-on-smart-contact-lenses-1405417127, 2014.

[6] International Organization for Standardization, ISO10993-1:2009. Biological evaluation of medical devices. Part 1: evaluation and testing within a risk management process, 2009.

[7] Evaluate, EvaluatedMedTech World Preview 2014, Outlook to 2020. Retrieved September 18, 2014, from http://www.evaluategroup.com/public/Reports/EvaluateMedTech-World-Preview-2014.aspx.

[8] Chameleon Pharma Consulting, Medical device market: the pulse of the developing healthcare industry, from http://www.chameleon-pharma.com/experience/medical-devices/.

[9] Espicom, The world Medical Market book 2013, from https://www.ic.gc.ca/eic/site/lsg-dsv.nsf/eng/h_hn01736.html#product, 2013.

[10] Consumer Healthcare, Who Tops in Having the Biggest Medical Devices Market in BRIC Countries, from http://www.consumer-healthcaretrends.com/2014/04/whotops-in-having-biggest-medical.html#.U8XrFbGoV5w.

[11] World Health Organization, World Health Statistics 2014 PartIII Global health indicators, from http://apps.who.int/iris/bitstream/10665/112738/1/9789240692671_eng.pdf?ua=1, 2014.

[12] World Health Organization, Life expectancy. Retrieved September 04, 2014, from http://www.who.int/gho/mortality_burden_disease/life_tables/situation_trends/en/, 2014.

[13] G. Shayne Cox, Case Histories and Problem Resolution (Chapter 17), Safety Evaluation of Medical Devices, second ed., The U.S. Marcel Dekker, New York, 2002.

[14] Tox Town, Phthalates. Retrieved September 04, 2014, from http://toxtown.nlm.nih.gov/text_version/chemicals.php?id=24, 2014.

[15] Sky News, PIP Breast Implant Boss Jean-Claude Mas Jailed. Retrieved August 30, 2014, from http://news.sky.com/story/1180207/pip-breast-implant-boss-jean-claude-mas-jailed, 2013.

[16] P.H. King, R.C. Fries, A.T. Johnson, Design of Biomedical Devices and Systems, third ed., CRC Press, Boca Raton, FL, 2014.

[17] Markets and Markets, Biomaterials Market [By Products (Polymers, Metals, Ceramics, Natural Biomaterials) & Applications (Cardiovascular, Orthopedic, Dental, Plastic Surgery, Wound Healing, Tissue Engineering, Ophthalmology, Neurology Disorders)]—Global Forecasts to 2017 from http://www.marketsandmarkets.com/Market-Reports/biomaterials-393.html.

[18] Saudi Food & Drug Authority, Case studies of medical devices adverse events, Section 5. Retrieved November 06, 2014, from http://old.sfda.gov.sa/NR/rdonlyres/FA6EA2E9-DB07-4B45-B948-190BB8497F45/1959/MedicalDevicecasestudies.pdf, 2009.

[19] World Health Organization, Medical device regulations: global overview and guiding principles, from http://whqlibdoc.who.int/publications/2003/9241546182.pdf, 2003.

[20] U.S. International Trade Commission, Medical Devices Industry Assessment. Retrieved September 11, 2014, from http://ita.doc.gov/td/health/medical%20device%20industry%20assessment%20final%20ii%203-24-10.pdf.

[21] World Health Organization, Lists of medical devices. Retrieved September 11, 2014, from http://www.who.int/gho/health_technologies/medical_devices/lists/en/, 2014.

[22] U.S. Food and Drug Administration, General controls for medical devices. Retrieved October 03, 2014, from http://www.fda.gov/MedicalDevices/DeviceRegulationandGuidance/Overview/GeneralandSpecialControls/ucm055910.htm#top, 2014.

[23] U.S. Food and Drug Administration, Regulatory controls. Retrieved August 15, 2014, from http://www.fda.gov/MedicalDevices/DeviceRegulationandGuidance/Overview/GeneralandSpecialControls/ucm2005378.htm, 2014.

[24] U.S. Food and Drug Administration, Class I/II Exemptions. Retrieved August 16, 2014, from http://www.fda.gov/MedicalDevices/DeviceRegulationandGuidance/Overview/ClassifyYourDevice/ucm051549.htm, 2014.

[25] U.S. Food and Drug Administration, Premarket Notification (510k). Retrieved September 12, 2014, from http://www.fda.gov/medicaldevices/deviceregulationandguidance/howtomarketyourdevice/premarketsubmissions/premarketnotification510k/default.htm, 2014.

[26] U.S. Food and Drug Administration, PMA Approvals. Retrieved September 05, 2014, from http://www.fda.gov/medicaldevices/productsandmedicalprocedures/deviceapprovalsandclearances/pmaapprovals/default.htm, 2014.

[27] D. O'Leary, Medical device classification. Retrieved January 12, 2015, from http://www.ombuenterprises.com/LibraryPDFs/Medical_Device_Classification.pdf.

[28] European Union, Countries. Retrieved January 07, 2015, from http://europa.eu/about-eu/countries/index_en.htm.

[29] J.J. Tobin, Global marketing authorisation of biomaterials and medical devices, in: S.F. Amato, R.M. Ezzell (Eds.), Regulatory Affairs for Biomaterials and Medical Devices, Woodhead Publishing, 2015, pp. 93–114 (Chapter 7).

[30] D.B. Kramer, S. Xu, A.S. Kesselheim, Regulation of medical devices in the United States and European Union, N. Engl. J. Med. 366 (2012) 848–855.

[31] C. Sorenson, M. Drummond, Improving medical device regulation: The United States and Europe in perspective, Milbank Q. 92 (2014) 114–150.

[32] European Commission, Regulatory framework. Retrieved September 04, 2014, from http://ec.europa.eu/health/medical-devices/regulatory-framework/index_en.htm.

[33] European Parliament, Amendments adopted by the European Parliament on 22 October 2013 on the proposal for a regulation of the European Parliament and of the Council on medical devices, and amending Directive 2001/83/EC, Regulation (EC)

No. 178/2002 and Regulation (EC) No. 1223/2009. Retrieved January 22, 2015, from http://www.europarl.europa.eu/sides/getDoc.do?type=TA&language=EN&reference=P7-TA-2013-428, 2013.
[34] N. Pelle, Medical devices need tighter regs—but how much tighter? Eng. Technol. 8 (2013).
[35] European Commission, Citizens' summary—EU proposal on medical devices, 2012
[36] A. Fouretier, D. Bertram, New regulations on medical devices in Europe: what to expect? Expert Rev. Med. Dev. 11 (2014) 351–359.
[37] J. Zhang, Chapter 8 - Chinese Regulatory Framework, in: R.C. Bairu (Ed.), Global Clinical Trials, Academic Press, San Diego, 2011, pp. 159–168.
[38] Y. Liu, M. Pecht, Overview of China's medical device market and government regulatory agencies, in: Materials & Processes for Medical Devices Conference, Minneapolis, Minnesota, USA, 2009, pp. 257–261.
[39] China Food and Drug Administration, Regulations for the supervision and administration of medical devices, 2000.
[40] S.J. Rizzi, N.A. Beaver, China publishes regulations on medical device GMPs and inspection requirements, FDIL's Update Mag. (2010).
[41] MWE China Law Office, China overhauls regulation on the medical device industry. http://wwwmwechinalawcom/news/2014/chinalawalert0414ahtm.
[42] The Central People's Government of People's Republic of China, 中华人民共和国国务院令 第276号, 2000. http://www.gov.cn/gongbao/content/2000/content_60576.htm.
[43] China Food and Drug Administration, 中华人民共和国国务院令 第650号, 2014. http://www.sda.gov.cn/WS01/CL0784/97814.html.
[44] EMERGO, New Chinese medical device, IVD regulations take effect in October 2014. Retrieved October 20, 2014, from http://www.emergogroup.com/blog/2014/08/new-chinese-medical-device-ivd-regulations-take-effect-october-2014, 2014.
[45] China Food and Drug Administration, 2014. 医疗器械注册管理办法 (国家食品药品监督管理总局令第4号). Retrieved September 02, 2014, from http://www.sfda.gov.cn/WS01/CL1101/103756.html.
[46] EMERGO, Global medical device industry outlook for 2015. Retrieved January 22, 2015, from www2.emergogroup.com/files/2015-emergo-group-medical-device-industry-survey.pdf, 2015.
[47] Pharmaceuticals and Medical Devices Agency, 2014. Regulatory system for medical devices in Japan. Retrieved October 15, 2014, from http://www.std.pmda.go.jp/stdDB/index_e.html.
[48] Australian Government Department of Health Therapeutic Goods Administration, Who we are & what we do. Retrieved December 15, 2014, from http://www.tga.gov.au/about/tga-who-we-are.htm#.VEtO_RYo-AQ, 2014.
[49] Australian Government Department of Health Therapeutic Goods Administration, The regulation of medical devices. Retrieved December 15, 2014, from http://www.tga.gov.au/newsroom/btn-devices-basics-regulation.htm#.VEtQtRYo-AQ, 2014.
[50] K.S. Saini, India: medical device regulatory system, Handbook of Medical Device Regulatory Affairs in Asia, Pan Stanford Publishing, Boca Raton, FL, 2013, pp. 341–364.
[51] J.L. Wong, P. Teysseyre, 10 - Fundamentals of medical device approval in the Asia Pacific region, in: S.F. Amato, R.M. Ezzell (Eds.), Regulatory Affairs for Biomaterials and Medical Devices, Woodhead Publishing, 2015, pp. 159–174.
[52] Health Science Authority, Regulatory Framework. Retrieved September 20, 2014, from http://www.hsa.gov.sg/content/hsa/en/Health_Products_Regulation/Medical_Devices/Overview/Regulatory_Framework.html.

[53] Health Science Authority, Medical Device Guidance GN-12: Guidance on Grouping of Medical Devices for Product Registration Retrieved January 07, 2015, from http://www.hsa.gov.sg/content/dam/HSA/HPRG/Medical_Devices/Overview_Framework_Policies/Guidances_for_Medical_Device_Registration/GN-12-R1_Guidance%20on%20Grouping%20of%20Medical%20Devices%20for%20Product%20Registration.pdf, 2011.

[54] V.R. Sastri, Regulations for medical devices and application to plastics suppliers: history and overview, in: V.R. Sastri (Ed.), Plastics in Medical Devices, second ed., William Andrew Publishing, Oxford, 2014, pp. 9–18 (Chapter 2).

[55] A. Goodall, G. Bos, ISO 13485: 2003 medical devices—quality management systems—requirements for regulatory purposes, Handbook of Medical Device Regulatory Affairs in Asia, CRC Press Taylor & Francis Group, Boca Raton, FL, 2013, pp. 125–143.

[56] U.S. Food and Drug Administration, Quality System (QS) Regulation/Medical Device Good Manufacturing Practices. Retrieved October 16, 2014, from http://www.fda.gov/medicaldevices/deviceregulationandguidance/postmarketrequirements/qualitysystemsregulations/, 2014.

[57] U.S. Food and Drug Administration, Medical Devices; Current Good Manufacturing Practice (CGMP) Final Rule; Quality System Regulation. Retrieved January 02, 2015, from http://www.fda.gov/medicaldevices/deviceregulationandguidance/post marketrequirements/qualitysystemsregulations/ucm230127.htm, 2014.

[58] U.S. Food and Drug Administration, medical device quality systems manual: a small entity compliance guide. Retrieved January 02, 2015, from http://www.gmp-compliance.org/guidemgr/files/mdqs.manual.pdf, 1996.

[59] B. Grace, What is in the QSR/GMP? IEEE Eng. Med. Biol. Mag. 23 (2004) 83–85.

[60] B. Grace, What is the QSR/GMP, and why should you care? Eng. Med. Biol. Mag. IEEE 23 (2004) 98–99.

[61] ICG International Certification Group, ISO13485:2003-Management System Certification for Medical Device Manufacturers. Retrieved July 28, 2014, from http://icg-certification.com/index.php?id=107.

[62] International Organization for Standardization, ISO/TR 10013:2001 Guideline for quality management system documentation, 2001.

[63] Inc. AQA Company, ISO 13485 & 21 CFR 820 Template Documentation Quality Manual, 34 Operational Procedures and 26 Forms. Retrieved December 29, 2014, from http://www.isoxp.com/10Products/ISO13485Docu.aspx.

[64] I. Abuhav, ISO 13485: A complete guide to quality management in the medical device industry, CRC Press Taylor & Francis Group, 2012.

[65] K. Sundström, Quality system requirements for documents, records and change control. Retrieved December 29, 2014, from http://www.uef.fi/documents/976466/1745345/06-20-sundstrom_qms_dm_rm_cm/027fbc74-2edf-4c57-9a4c-581168468cf7, 2013.

[66] Praxiom Research Group Limited, ISO 13485 2003 Translated into Plain English. Retrieved December 29, 2014, from http://www.praxiom.com/iso-13485.htm, 2014.

[67] DITEK Corporation Inc., Quality management systems manual. Retrieved December 29, 2014, from http://www.ditekmfg.com/pdf/Ditek_QMS-Manual.pdf, 2011.

[68] E. Jeremy, Implementing an ISO13485 Medical Devices Quality Management System. Retrieved December 29, 2014, from http://www.asqlongisland.org/seminars/Implementing_13485.pdf.

[69] I.H. Abdul Razak, S. Kamaruddin, I. Abdul Azid, I. Putra Almanar, ISO 13485: 2003: implementation reference model from the Malaysian SMEs medical device industry, TQM J. 21 (2009) 6–19.

[70] International Organization for Standardization, Medical devices-quality management systems-guidance on the application of ISO 13485:2003, 2005.
[71] J. Chai, Regulation of medical devices in the European Union, J. Leg. Med. 21 (2000) 537–556.
[72] E. French-Mowat, J. Burnett, How are medical devices regulated in the European Union? J. R. Soc. Med. 105 (Suppl. 1) (2012) S22–S28.
[73] EMERGO, ISO 13485 Consulting and Implementation for Medical Device Manufacturers. Retrieved January 11, 2015, from http://www.emergogroup.com/services/worldwide/iso-13485-consulting, 2015.
[74] TÜV SÜD, ISO 13485 Quality Management System for Medical Devices. Retrieved January 11, 2015, from http://www.tuv-sud.com/industry/healthcare-medical-device/quality-management-quality-control-for-medical-devices/iso-13485-quality-management-system-for-medical-devices#tab_1397654991943280823715.
[75] EMERGO, Japan PMDL Quality Management System Compliance - MHLW Ordinance #169. Retrieved January 11, 2015, from http://www.emergogroup.com/services/japan/quality-system-compliance-japan, 2015.
[76] Pharmaceuticals and Medical Devices Agency Office of GMP/QMS Inspection, Current situation and updates of QMS inspection in Japan. Retrieved January 11, 2015, from http://www.pmda.go.jp/regulatory/file/english_presentation/GMP_QMS/G-E2makino.pdf.
[77] International Organization for Standardization, ISO14971:2012 Medical devices—application of risk management to medical devices, 2012.
[78] International Organization for Standardization, ISO/TR 14969:2005 Medical devices—quality management systems—guidance on the application of ISO13485:2003, 2005.
[79] U S Food and Drug Administration, Facts About the Current Good Manufacturing Practices (CGMPs). Retrieved October 03, 2014, from http://www.fda.gov/Drugs/Development ApprovalProcess/Manufacturing/ucm169105.htm, 2015.
[80] C. George, An overview of a medical device quality system. Retrieved January 11, 2015, from http://www.regdesk.co/Blog/Blog8, 2014.
[81] S.F. Amato, 3 - Regulatory strategies for biomaterials and medical devices in the USA: classification, design, and risk analysis, in: S.F. Amato, R.M. Ezzell (Eds.), Regulatory Affairs for Biomaterials and Medical Devices, Woodhead Publishing, 2015, pp. 27–46.
[82] Betty Lane, Overview of ISO 13485—Medical Device Quality Management System Requirements. Retrieved August 15, 2015, from http://www.mastercontrol.com/newsletter/medical_device/iso_13485_overview_0110.html.
[83] BNP Media Staff, ISO 13485: Just the facts. Retrieved October 09, 2014, from http://www.qualitymag.com/articles/86067-iso-13485-just-the-facts, 2008.
[84] U.S. Food and Drug Administration, Product classification. Retrieved December 12, 2014, from http://www.accessdata.fda.gov/scripts/cdrh/cfdocs/cfpcd/classification.cfm.
[85] U.S. Food and Drug Administration, Classify your medical device. Retrieved December 23, 2014, from http://www.fda.gov/MedicalDevices/DeviceRegulationandGuidance/Overview/ClassifyYourDevice/default.htm.
[86] U.S. Food and Drug Administration, 510(k) submission methods. Retrieved January 14, 2015, from http://www.fda.gov/MedicalDevices/DeviceRegulationandGuidance/HowtoMarketYourDevice/PremarketSubmissions/PremarketNotification510k/ucm134034.htm, 2014.
[87] U.S. Food and Drug Administration, Evaluation of automatic class III designation (De Novo) summaries. Retrieved January 14, 2015, from http://www.fda.gov/AboutFDA/CentersOffices/OfficeofMedicalProductsandTobacco/CDRH/CDRHTransparency/ucm232269.htm.

[88] U.S. Food and Drug Administration, PMA application methods. Retrieved January 14, 2015, from http://www.fda.gov/MedicalDevices/DeviceRegulationandGuidance/HowtoMarketYourDevice/PremarketSubmissions/PremarketApprovalPMA/ucm048168.htm, 2014.
[89] U.S. Food and Drug Administration, Content of a 510(k). Retrieved January 05, 2015, from http://www.fda.gov/MedicalDevices/DeviceRegulationandGuidance/HowtoMarketYourDevice/PremarketSubmissions/PremarketNotification510k/ucm142651.htm, 2014.
[90] U.S. Food and Drug Administration, Guidance for industry and FDA staff: format for traditional and abbreviated 510(k)s. Retrieved January 16, 2015, from http://www.fda.gov/MedicalDevices/DeviceRegulationandGuidance/GuidanceDocuments/ucm084365.htm, 2005.
[91] U.S. Food and Drug Administration, CFR—Code of Federal Regulations Title 21 Part 807 Establishment Registration and Device Listing for Manufacturers and Initial Importers of Devices. Retrieved December 24, 2014, from http://www.accessdata.fda.gov/scripts/cdrh/cfdocs/cfcfr/CFRSearch.cfm?CFRPart=807&showFR=1&subpartNode=21:8.0.1.1.5.5, 2014.
[92] U.S. Food and Drug Administration, User fee system. Retrieved January 05, 2015, from https://userfees.fda.gov/mdufa.
[93] U.S. Food and Drug Administration, Medical device user fees for fiscal year 2015 (October 1, 2014 - September 30, 2015). Retrieved January 07, 2015, from http://www.fda.gov/MedicalDevices/ResourcesforYou/Industry/ucm407660.htm, 2015.
[94] U.S. Food and Drug Administration, MDUFMA user fees cover sheet. Retrieved January 07, 2015, from http://www.fda.gov/ForIndustry/UserFees/MedicalDeviceUserFeeandModernizationAct/ucm155274.htm, 2014.
[95] U.S. Food and Drug Administration, Current list of accredited persons for 510(k) review under the FDA Modernization Act of 1997. Retrieved January 29, 2015, from http://www.accessdata.fda.gov/scripts/cdrh/cfdocs/cfthirdparty/accredit.cfm, 2015.
[96] U.S. Food and Drug Administration, List of Devices for Third Party Review. Retrieved January 29, 2015, from http://www.accessdata.fda.gov/scripts/cdrh/cfdocs/cfThirdParty/current.cfm#1, 2002.
[97] U.S. Food and Drug Administration, Third party review. Retrieved January 29, 2015, from http://www.fda.gov/medicaldevices/deviceregulationandguidance/howtomarketyourdevice/premarketsubmissions/thirdparyreview/default.htm, 2014.
[98] U.S. Food and Drug Administration, Implementation of third party programs under the FDA Modernization Act of 1997; final guidance for staff, industry and third parties. Retrieved January 29, 2015, from http://www.fda.gov/MedicalDevices/DeviceRegulationandGuidance/GuidanceDocuments/ucm094450.htm, 2001.
[99] U.S. Food and Drug Administration, Acceptance Checklist for 510(k)s. Retrieved January 06, 2015, from http://www.fda.gov/MedicalDevices/DeviceRegulationandGuidance/HowtoMarketYourDevice/PremarketSubmissions/PremarketNotification510k/ucm 071360.htm, 2013.
[100] U.S. Food and Drug Administration, Indications for use statement. Retrieved January 07, 2015, from http://www.fda.gov/MedicalDevices/DeviceRegulationandGuidance/GuidanceDocuments/ucm080275.htm, 2014.
[101] U.S. Food and Drug Administration, CFR—Code of Federal Regulations Title 21. Retrieved January 07, 2015, from http://www.accessdata.fda.gov/scripts/cdrh/cfdocs/cfCFR/CFRSearch.cfm?FR=807.92, 2014.
[102] U S Food and Drug Administration, The 510(k) program: evaluating substantial equivalence in premarket notifications [510(k)]—guidance for Industry and Food and Drug

Administration Staff. Retrieved January 07, 2015, from http://www.fda.gov/downloads/MedicalDevices/DeviceRegulationandGuidance/GuidanceDocuments/UCM284443.pdf, 2014.

[103] U.S. Food and Drug Administration, CFR - Code of Federal Regulations Title 21—21CFR807.93. Retrieved January 08, 2015, from http://www.accessdata.fda.gov/scripts/cdrh/cfdocs/cfCFR/CFRSearch.cfm?FR=807.93, 2014.

[104] U.S. Food and Drug Administration, Premarket Notification 510(k) Statement. Retrieved January 06, 2015, from http://www.fda.gov/MedicalDevices/DeviceRegulationandGuidance/HowtoMarketYourDevice/PremarketSubmissions/PremarketNotification510k/ucm142664.htm, 2009.

[105] U.S. Food and Drug Administration, Premarket notification truthful and accurate statement. Retrieved January 06, 2015, from http://www.fda.gov/MedicalDevices/DeviceRegulationandGuidance/HowtoMarketYourDevice/PremarketSubmissions/PremarketNotification510k/ucm142707.htm, 2009.

[106] U.S. Food and Drug Administration, Premarket notification Class III certification and summary. Retrieved January 16, 2015, from http://www.fda.gov/MedicalDevices/Device RegulationandGuidance/HowtoMarketYourDevice/PremarketSubmissions/PremarketNotification510k/ucm142662.htm.

[107] U.S. Food and Drug Administration, Guidance for Industry and FDA Staff - Recognition and Use of Consensus Standards. Retrieved January 16, 2015, from http://www.fda.gov/MedicalDevices/DeviceRegulationandGuidance/GuidanceDocuments/ucm077274.htm, 2007.

[108] U.S. Food and Drug Administration, Guidance for industry and for FDA staff: use of standards in substantial equivalence determinations. Retrieved January 16, 2015, from http://www.fda.gov/MedicalDevices/DeviceRegulationandGuidance/GuidanceDocuments/ucm073752.htm, 2000.

[109] U.S. Food and Drug Administration, An innovative "Me-Too" Idea: Premarket Notification—510(k) medical device submissions: instructor's guide. Retrieved October 20, 2014, from www.fda.gov/downloads/Training/CourseMaterialsforEducators/NationalMedicalDeviceCurriculum/UCM406370.pdf, 2014.

[110] U.S. Food and Drug Administration, CFR - Code of Federal Regulations Title 21 PART 801 LABELING. Retrieved January 08, 2015, from http://www.accessdata.fda.gov/scripts/cdrh/cfdocs/cfCFR/CFRSearch.cfm?CFRPart=801, 2014.

[111] U.S. Food and Drug Administration, Device Labeling Guidance #G91-1 (blue book memo) (Text Only). Retrieved January 20, 2015, from http://www.fda.gov/MedicalDevices/DeviceRegulationandGuidance/GuidanceDocuments/ucm081368.htm, 2014.

[112] U.S. Food and Drug Administration, Guidance Documents (Medical Devices and Radiation-Emitting Products). Retrieved January 30, 2015, from http://www.fda.gov/MedicalDevices/DeviceRegulationandGuidance/GuidanceDocuments/default.htm, 2015.

[113] U.S. Food and Drug Administration, Recognized Consensus Standards, from http://www.accessdata.fda.gov/scripts/cdrh/cfdocs/cfstandards/search.cfm, 2013.

[114] U.S. Food and Drug Administration, Deciding When to Submit a 510(k) for a Change to an Existing Device (K97-1). Retrieved January 22, 2015, from http://www.fda.gov/MedicalDevices/DeviceRegulationandGuidance/GuidanceDocuments/ucm080235.htm, 1997.

[115] U.S. Food and Drug Administration, Required Elements for a Declaration of Conformity to a Recognized Standard. Retrieved January 22, 2015, from http://www.fda.gov/MedicalDevices/DeviceRegulationandGuidance/HowtoMarketYourDevice/Premarket Submissions/PremarketNotification510k/ucm142706.htm, 2009.

[116] U.S. Food and Drug Administration, How To Prepare A Special 510(k). Retrieved January 22, 2015, from http://www.fda.gov/MedicalDevices/DeviceRegulationandGuidance/HowtoMarketYourDevice/PremarketSubmissions/PremarketNotification510k/ucm134573.htm, 2014.

[117] U.S. Food and Drug Administration, Case study—a fledgling company works to bring its first product to market-Regulatory pathways for medical devices: choosing the right one. Retrieved October 20, 2014, from http://www.fda.gov/downloads/Training/CourseMaterialsforEducators/NationalMedicalDeviceCurriculum/UCM404247.pdf, 2014.

[118] U.S. Food and Drug Administration, CFR—Code of Federal Regulations Title 21 part 814premarket approval of medical devices. Retrieved January 08, 2015, from http://www.accessdata.fda.gov/scripts/cdrh/cfdocs/cfcfr/CFRSearch.cfm?CFRPart=814&showFR=1, 2014.

[119] U.S. Food and Drug Administration, PMA application contents. Retrieved January 08, 2015, from http://www.fda.gov/MedicalDevices/DeviceRegulationandGuidance/HowtoMarketYourDevice/PremarketSubmissions/PremarketApprovalPMA/ucm050289.htm, 2014.

[120] U.S. Food and Drug Administration, CFR - Code of Federal Regulations Title 21860.7 Determination of safety and effectiveness. Retrieved January 23, 2015, from http://www.accessdata.fda.gov/scripts/cdrh/cfdocs/cfcfr/CFRSearch.cfm?FR=860.7, 2014.

[121] U.S. Food and Drug Administration, CFR - Code of Federal Regulations Title 21 PART 898 performance standard for electrode lead wires and patient cables. Retrieved January 23, 2015, from http://www.accessdata.fda.gov/scripts/cdrh/cfdocs/cfcfr/CFRSearch.cfm?CFRPart=898, 2014.

[122] U.S. Food and Drug Administration, Performance Standards. Retrieved January 23, 2015, from http://www.fda.gov/Radiation-EmittingProducts/ElectronicProductRadiationControlProgram/GettingaProducttoMarket/PerformanceStandards/default.htm, 2014.

[123] U.S. Food and Drug Administration, CFR—Code of Federal Regulations Title 21 part 58 good laboratory practice for nonclinical laboratory studies. Retrieved January 23, 2015, from http://www.accessdata.fda.gov/scripts/cdrh/cfdocs/cfcfr/CFRSearch.cfm?CFRPart=58&showFR=1, 2014.

[124] U.S. Food and Drug Administration, CFR—Code of Federal Regulations Title 21 part 56 institutional review boards. Retrieved January 23, 2015, from http://www.accessdata.fda.gov/scripts/cdrh/cfdocs/cfcfr/CFRSearch.cfm?CFRPart=56&showFR=1, 2014.

[125] U.S. Food and Drug Administration CFR—code of federal regulations title 21 part 56 institutional review boards. Retrieved January 23, 2015, from http://www.accessdata.fda.gov/scripts/cdrh/cfdocs/cfcfr/CFRSearch.cfm?CFRPart=56&showFR=1, 2014.

[126] U.S. Food and drug administration, CFR—Code of Federal Regulations Title 21 Part 812 investigational device exemptions. Retrieved January 23, 2015, from http://www.accessdata.fda.gov/scripts/cdrh/cfdocs/cfcfr/CFRSearch.cfm?CFRPart=812, 2014.

[127] U.S. Food and Drug Administration, PMA labeling. Retrieved January 23, 2015, from http://www.fda.gov/medicaldevices/deviceregulationandguidance/howtomarketyourdevice/premarketsubmissions/premarketapprovalpma/ucm050390.htm, 2014.

[128] U.S. Food and Drug Administration, CFR - Code of Federal Regulations Title 21 Part 25 enviromental impact considerations. Retrieved January 23, 2015, from http://www.accessdata.fda.gov/scripts/cdrh/cfdocs/cfcfr/CFRSearch.cfm?CFRPart=25.

[129] U.S. Food and Drug Administration, CFR—Code of Federal Regulations Title 21 Part 54 Financial Disclosure by Clinical Investigators. Retrieved January 23, 2015, from http://www.accessdata.fda.gov/scripts/cdrh/cfdocs/cfcfr/CFRSearch.cfm?CFRPart=54, 2014.

[130] U.S. Food and Drug Administration, IDE application. Retrieved January 08, 2015, from http://www.fda.gov/MedicalDevices/DeviceRegulationandGuidance/HowtoMarketYourDevice/InvestigationalDeviceExemptionIDE/ucm046706.htm, 2014.

[131] ClinicalTrials.gov—a service of the U.S. National Institues of Health. Retrieved January 26, 2015, from https://www.clinicaltrials.gov/.

[132] U.S. Food and Drug Administration, eCopy Program for Medical Device Submissions. Retrieved January 26, 2015, from http://www.fda.gov/MedicalDevices/DeviceRegulationandGuidance/HowtoMarketYourDevice/ucm370879.htm, 2014.

[133] U.S. Food and Drug Administration, FY 2015 Medical Device User Fee Small Business Qualification and Certification Guidance for Industry, Food and Drug Administration Staff and Foreign Governments. Retrieved October 20, 2014, from http://www.fda.gov/downloads/MedicalDevices/DeviceRegulationandGuidance/Overview/MDUFAIII/UCM314389.pdf, 2014.

[134] U.S. Food and Drug Administration, 510(k) Submission process. Retrieved January 26, 2015, from http://www.fda.gov/MedicalDevices/DeviceRegulationandGuidance/HowtoMarketYourDevice/PremarketSubmissions/PremarketNotification510k/ucm070201.htm, 2014.

[135] U.S. Food and Drug Administration, Federal Food, Drug, and Cosmetic Act (FD&C) Sec. 515(c)(1). Application for Premarket Approval. Retrieved January 28, 2015, from http://www.gpo.gov/fdsys/pkg/USCODE-2010-title21/pdf/USCODE-2010-title21-chap9-subchapV-partA-sec360e.pdf, 1997.

[136] U.S. Food and Drug Administration, CFR—Code of Federal Regulations Title 21 Part 814 —Premarket Approval of Medical Devices Retrieved Januray 08, 2015, from http://www.accessdata.fda.gov/scripts/cdrh/cfdocs/cfcfr/CFRSearch.cfm?FR=814.20, 2014.

[137] U.S. Food and Drug Administration, Premarket Approval Application Modular Review. Retrieved January 29, 2015, from http://www.fda.gov/MedicalDevices/DeviceRegulationandGuidance/GuidanceDocuments/ucm089764.htm, 2003.

[138] U.S. Food and Drug Administration, FDA Industry Systems. Retrieved January 26, 2015, from https://www.access.fda.gov/oaa/logonFlow.htm?execution=e1s1.

[139] U.S. Food and Drug Administration, Device facility user fee website. Retrieved January 26, 2015, from https://userfees.fda.gov/OA_HTML/furls.jsp.

[140] EMERGO, Europe CE approval process for medical devices. Retrieved October 21, 2014, from http://www.emergogroup.com/resources/europe-process-chart, 2013.

[141] S. Zhang, C. Kriza, P.L. Kolominsky-Rabas, Assessing new developments in the pre-market regulatory process of medical devices in the People's Republic of China, Expert Rev. Med. Dev. 11 (2014) 527–535.

[142] China Food and Drug Administration, 食品药品监管总局办公厅关于实施第一类医疗器械备案有关事项的通知. Retrieved January 13, 2015, from http://www.sfda.gov.cn/WS01/CL1105/106435.html, 2014.

[143] China Food and Drug Administration, 境内第二类医疗器械注册审批操作规范. Retrieved September 02, 2014, from http://www.sfda.gov.cn/WS01/CL1105/106258.html, 2014.

[144] China Food and Drug Administration, 境内第三类和进口医疗器械注册审批操作规范. Retrieved September 02, 2014, from http://www.sfda.gov.cn/WS01/CL1105/106257.html, 2014.

[145] China Food and Drug Administration, 境内医疗器械注册申请表. Retrieved January 18, 2015, from http://www.sfda.gov.cn/WS01/CL0029/108402.html, 2014.

[146] China Food and Drug Administration, 进口医疗器械注册申请表. Retrieved January 18, 2015, from http://www.sfda.gov.cn/WS01/CL0029/108394.html, 2014.
[147] Health Science Authority, Quick guide to medical device product registration and licensing. Retrieved October 05, 2014, from http://www.hsa.gov.sg/content/dam/HSA/HPRG/Medical_Devices/Overview_Framework_Policies/Regulatory_Framework/QUICK%20GUIDE%20TO%20MEDICAL%20DEVICE%20PRODUCT%20REGISTRATION%20AND%20LICENSING%20%28WORD%29_13%20Dec%202010_Ver.1.pdf
[148] ASEAN Consultative Committee for Standards & Quality Medical Device Product Working Group, Common Submission Dossier Template. Retrieved January 13, 2015, from http://www.asean.org/archive/SnC/ASEAN%20MDPWG%20CSDT_Final_21%20Oct%202010.pdf, 2010.
[149] Health Science Authority, MEDICAL DEVICE GUIDANCE-GN-17: Guidance on Preparation of a Product Registration Submission for General Medical Devices using the ASEAN CSDT. Retrieved January 13, 2015, from http://www.hsa.gov.sg/content/dam/HSA/HPRG/Medical_Devices/Overview_Framework_Policies/Guidances_for_Medical_Device_Registration/GN-17-D1.1%20Guidance%20on%20Preparation%20of%20a%20Product%20Registration%20Submission%20for%20GMD%20using%20the%20ASEAN%20CSDT.pdf, 2014.
[150] Health Science Authority, Target processing timelines. Retrieved October 17, 2014, from http://www.hsa.gov.sg/content/hsa/en/Health_Products_Regulation/Medical_Devices/Application_Registration/Target_Processing_Timelines.html, 2014.
[151] Health Science Authority, Fees and Charges. Retrieved August 28, 2014, from http://www.hsa.gov.sg/content/hsa/en/Health_Products_Regulation/Medical_Devices/Application_Registration/Fees_and_Charges.html, 2014.
[152] International Electrotechnical Commission, IEC 60601-1 Medical electrical equipment–Part 1: General requirements for basic safety and essential performance, from http://webstore.iec.ch/preview/info_iec60601-1%7Bed3.1%7Den.pdf, 2012.
[153] International Electrotechnical Commission, IEC 60601-1-2 ed4.0 Medical electrical equipment—Part 1-2: general requirements for basic safety and essential performance—collateral standard: electromagnetic disturbances—requirements and tests, 2014.
[154] International Electrotechnical Commission, IEC61025 Fault tree analysis (FTA), from http://webstore.iec.ch/preview/info_iec61025%7Bed2.0%7Den_d.pdf, 2006.
[155] W.A. Hyman, E. Johnson, Fault tree analysis of clinical alarms, J. Clin. Eng. 33 (2008) 85–94, http://dx.doi.org/10.1097/01.JCE.0000305872.86942.66.
[156] Organisation for Economic Co-operation and Development, OECD Guideline for the Testing of Chemicals. In vitro mammalian cell gene mutation test, 1997.
[157] Organisation for Economic Co-operation and Development, OECD Guideline for the Testing of Chemicals. Carcinogenicity Studies, from http://www.oecd.org/chemicalsafety/testing/41753121.pdf, 2008.
[158] Organisation for Economic Co-operation and Development, OECD Guideline for the Testing of Chemicals. Reproduction/Developmental Toxicity Screening Test, from http://ntp.niehs.nih.gov/iccvam/suppdocs/feddocs/oecd/oecd_gl421.pdf, 1995.
[159] International Organization of Standardization, ISO 10993–6:2007 Biological evaluation of medical devices—part 6: tests for local effects after implantation, 2007.
[160] International Organization of Standardization, ISO 10993-4:2002 Biological evaluation of medical devices—part 4: selection of tests for interactions with blood, 2002.
[161] S Food and Drug Administration, Updated 510(k) Sterility Review Guidance K90-1; Guidance for Industry and FDA, from http://www.fda.gov/downloads/MedicalDevices/DeviceRegulationandGuidance/GuidanceDocuments/ucm072790.pdf, 2002.

[162] International Safety Transit Association. Retrieved from http://www.ista.org/.

[163] ASTM International, ASTM D4169-14, Standard practice for performance testing of shipping containers and systems. West Conshohocken, PA, 2014.

[164] European Commission, MEDICAL DEVICES : Guidance document MEDDEV 2. 2/1 Rev1-GUIDELINES RELATING TO THE APPLICATION OF : THE COUNCIL DIRECTIVE 90/385/EEC ON ACTIVE IMPLANTABLE MEDICAL DEVICES THE COUNCIL DIRECTIVE 93/42/EEC ON MEDICAL DEVICES, from http://ec.europa.eu/health/medical-devices/files/meddev/2_2-1____02-1998_en.pdf, 1998.

[165] G. Shayne Cox, Clinical studies for medical devices, Safety Evaluation of Medical Devices, second ed., Marcel Dekker, USA, 2002 (Chapter 15).

[166] U.S. Food and Drug Administration, Case Study A stent company seeks to market a novel medical device-Bringing an innovative device to market: premarket approval (PMA) of medical devices. Retrieved November 05, 2014, from http://www.fda.gov/downloads/aboutfda/reportsmanualsforms/forms/ucm404249.pdf, 2014.

[167] U.S. Food and Drug Administration, Conducting Clinical Trials. Retrieved September 17, 2014, from http://www.fda.gov/drugs/developmentapprovalprocess/conductingclinicaltrials/default.htm, 2014.

[168] Duncan Fatz, Guide to European Medical Device Trials and BS EN ISO 14155. UK: BSI Standards Limited; 2012.

[169] Medicines and Healthcare products Regulatory Agency, Clinical investigations of medical devices-guidance for manufacturers Retrieved October 09, 2014, from http://www.mhra.gov.uk/home/groups/es-era/documents/publication/con007504.pdf, 2013.

[170] European Commission, MEDDEV.2.7.1 Rev.3 clinical evaluation: a guide for manufacturers and notified bodies, from http://ec.europa.eu/health/medical-devices/files/meddev/2_7_1rev_3_en.pdf, 2009.

[171] Microsoft, Test your document's readability Retrieved September 30, 2014, from http://office.microsoft.com/en-sg/word-help/test-your-document-s-readability-HP010148506.aspx.

[172] S. Mehta Shreefal, Commericializing Successful Biomedical Technologies-Basic Principles for the Development of Drugs, Diagnostics and Devices, U.S Cambridge University Press, 2008.

[173] International Organization of Standardization, ISO14155:2011 Clinical investigation of medical devices for human subjects—good clinical practice, 2011.

[174] U.S. Food and Drug Administration, Informed Consent Information Sheet Guidance for IRBs, Clinical Investigators, and Sponsors (draft guidance). Retrieved November 05, 2014, from http://www.fda.gov/downloads/aboutfda/reportsmanualsforms/forms/ucm405006.pdf, 2014.

[175] World Medical Association, WMA Declaration of Helsinki-Ethical Principles for Medical Research Involving Human Subjects. Retrieved September 24, 2014, from http://www.wma.net/en/30publications/10policies/b3/.

[176] ClinicalTrials.gov, History, Policies, and Laws. Retrieved September 24, 2014.

[177] U.S. Food and Drug Administration Center for Devices and Radiological Health, Good Clinical Practice 101: An Introduction Retrieved October 24, 2014, from http://fda.yorkcast.com/webcast/Play/477af877491747379c36c4ab1c7421b9, 2009.

[178] Division of Microbiology and Infectious Diseases (DMID), National Institute of Allergy and Infectious Diseases (NIAID), National Institutes of Health (NIH), Good Clinical Practice Resource Guide, from http://www.niaid.nih.gov/LabsAndResources/resources/DMIDClin Rsrch/Documents/handbook.pdf, 2011.

[179] National Institute of Allergy and Infectious Disease Division of Microbiology and Infectious Diseases, Good Clinical Practise Researces Guide, from http://www.niaid.nih.gov/labsandresources/resources/dmidclinrsrch/documents/handbook.pdf, 2011.

[180] F. Parquin, A. Audry, Clinical evaluation of medical devices: main constraints and specificities, Therapie 67 (2012) 311–318.

[181] D.A. Zarin, A. Keselman, Registering a clinical trial in ClinicalTrials.gov, Chest 131 (2007) 909–912.

[182] T. Tse, R.J. Williams, D.A. Zarin, Reporting 'basic results' in ClinicalTrials.gov, Chest 136 (2009) 295–303.

[183] U.S. Food and Drug Administration, Certifications To Accompany Drug, Biological Product, and Device Applications/Submissions: Compliance with Section 402(j) of The Public Health Service Act, Added By Title VIII of The Food and Drug Administration Amendments Act of 2007 Guidance for Sponsors, Industry, Researchers, Investigators, and Food and Drug Administration Staff, from http://www.fda.gov/RegulatoryInformation/Guidances/ucm125335.htm, 2009.

[184] U.S. Food and Drug Administration, Certification of compliance. Retrieved September 24, 2015, from http://www.fda.gov/downloads/aboutfda/reportsmanualsforms/forms/ucm048364.pdf.

[185] U.S. Food and Drug Administration, INstructions For Completion Of Form FDA 3674—Certification of compliance Under 42 U.S.C. § 282(j)(5)(B), with Requirements of ClinicalTrials.gov Data Bank (42 U.S.C. § 282(j)) from http://www.fda.gov/downloads/aboutfda/reportsmanualsforms/forms/ucm354618.pdf.

[186] U.S. Food and Drug Administration, The Sponsor: Responsibilities in Medical Device Clinical Trials Retrieved October 24, 2014, from http://fda.yorkcast.com/webcast/Play/88f92205e9624bbea1d627126af5360f, 2009.

[187] U.S. Food and Drug Administration, The Clinical Investigator: Responsibilities in Medical Device Trials. Retrieved October 24, 2014, from http://fda.yorkcast.com/webcast/Play/29b55c1dd3f64d8fa74ca2227df14b39, 2009.

[188] National Healthcare Group, Singapore Guideline for Good Clinical Practice Course. Retrieved September 25, 2014, from https://www.research.nhg.com.sg/wps/wcm/connect/romp/nhgromp/trainingeducation/coursecategories/singapore+guideline+for+good+clinical+practice+course.

[189] Medicines and Healthcare products Regulatory Agency, Clinical investigations of medial devices-statistical considerations. Retrieved October 09, 2014, from http://www.mhra.gov.uk/home/groups/es-era/documents/publication/con007518.pdf, 2013.

[190] Medical University of Vienna, Clinical Investigation Plan, from http://www.meduniwien.ac.at/hp/1/kks/partner-links-downloads/downloads/.

[191] Irish Clinical Research Infrastructure Network, Template Clinical Investigation Report, from http://www.molecularmedicineireland.ie/uploads/MMIICRIN-CIR%20Template-updateddec2013.pdf.

[192] U.S. Food and Drug Administration, MAUDE—Manufacturer and User Facility Device Experience. Retrieved Oct-14, 2014, from http://www.accessdata.fda.gov/scripts/cdrh/cfdocs/cfMAUDE/search.CFM, 2014.

[193] Medicines and Healthcare products Regulatory Agency, Clinical investigations of medical devices-guidance for pre-clinical assessors, Retrieved October 14, 2014, from http://www.mhra.gov.uk/home/groups/es-era/documents/publication/con007508.pdf, 2013.

[194] P.K. Drain, M. Robine, K.K. Holmes, I.V. Bassett, Trail watch: global migration of clinical trials, Nat. Rev. Drug Discov. 13 (2014) 166–167.

[195] G. Minisman, M. Bhanushali, R. Conwit, G.I. Wolfe, I. Aban, H.J. Kaminski, et al., Implementing clinical trials on an international platform: challenges and perspectives, J. Neurol. Sci. 313 (2012) 1–6.
[196] U.S. Food and Drug Administration, Case study-Regulatory pathways for pediatric medical devices: marketing a pediatric medical device via a humanitarian device exemption. Retrieved October 27, 2014, from http://www.fda.gov/downloads/Training/CourseMaterialsforEducators/NationalMedicalDeviceCurriculum/UCM416712.pdf, 2014.
[197] M.C. Luke, Regulatory Challenges in Extrapolation of Adult Medical Device Data to Pediatric Populations. Retrieved October 27, 2014, from http://www.fda.gov/downloads/MedicalDevices/NewsEvents/WorkshopsConferences/UCM285293.pdf.
[198] G. SeowLi-Ping, Regulatory Affairs for Medical Device Clinical Trials in Asia Pacific, Handbook of Medical Device Regulatory Affairs in Asia, Pan Stanford Publishing, 2013.
[199] Inc. Association for the Accreditation of Human Research Protection Programs. Accredited Organizations. Retrieved January 13, 2015, from http://www.aahrpp.org/learn/find-an-accredited-organization.
[200] Y. Sato, K. Koyama, Clinical research in Japan: past, present and future, Keio J. Med. 59 (2010) 104–109.
[201] U.S. Food and Drug Administration, Design Control Guidance For Medical Device Manufacturers, from http://www.fda.gov/MedicalDevices/DeviceRegulationandGuidance/GuidanceDocuments/ucm070627.htm#_Toc382720787, 2014.
[202] Department of Health and Human Services (USA), Investigational devices: four case studies. Retrieved October 07, 2014, from https://oig.hhs.gov/oei/reports/oei-05-94-00100.pdf, 1995.
[203] U.S. Food and Drug Administration, National Medical Device Curriculum. Retrieved October 16, 2014, from http://www.fda.gov/Training/CourseMaterialsforEducators/National MedicalDeviceCurriculum/ucm404244.htm.
[204] U.S. Food and Drug Administration, Case studies. Retrieved October 16, 2014, from http://www.fda.gov/Training/CourseMaterialsforEducators/NationalMedicalDeviceCurriculum/ucm404245.htm#c3, 2014.
[205] U.S. Food and Drug Administration, Questions and answers about eMDR—electronic medical device reporting—guidance for industry, user facilities and FDA staff. Retrieved October 16, 2015, from http://www.fda.gov/MedicalDevices/DeviceRegulationandGuidance/GuidanceDocuments/ucm175805.htm, 2014.
[206] U.S. Food and Drug Administration, Learn if a medical device has been cleared by FDA for marketing. Retrieved October 10, 2014, from http://www.fda.gov/MedicalDevices/ResourcesforYou/Consumers/ucm142523.htm, 2014.
[207] C.T. DeMarco, Medical Device Design and Regulation, ASQ Quality Press, 2011.
[208] M. Perán, M. García, E. Lopez-Ruiz, G. Jiménez, J. Marchal, How can nanotechnology help to repair the body? Advances in cardiac, skin, bone, cartilage and nerve tissue regeneration, Materials 6 (2013) 1333–1359.
[209] J. Paradise, A.W. Tisdale, R.F. Hall, E. Kokkoli, Evaluating oversight of human drugs and medical devices: a case study of the FDA and implications for nanobiotechnology, J. Law Med. Ethics 37 (2009) 598–624.
[210] U.S. Food and Drug Administration, Nanotechnology—a report of the U.S. Food and Drug Administration Nanotechnology Task Force. Retrieved October 10, 2014, from http://www.fda.gov/downloads/ScienceResearch/SpecialTopics/Nanotechnology/ucm110856.pdf, 2007.

[211] S.B. Foote, Commentary: evaluating oversight of human drugs and medical devices, J. Law Med. Ethics 37 (2009) 629–632.
[212] J. Paradise, S.M. Wolf, J. Kuzma, A. Kuzhabekova, A.W. Tisdale, E. Kokkoli, et al., Developing U.S. oversight strategies for nanobiotechnology: learning from past oversight experiences, J. Law Med. Ethics 37 (2009) 688–705.
[213] U.S. Food and Drug Administration, Guidance for industry considering whether an FDA-regulated product involves the application of nanotechnology. Retrieved October 14, 2014, from http://www.fda.gov/downloads/RegulatoryInformation/Guidances/UCM401695.pdf, 2014.
[214] United Kingdom Royal Society, Nanoscience and nanotechnologies: opportunities and uncertainties. Retrieved October 14, 2014, 2004.
[215] V. Gill, Nano-regulation creeps closer. Retrieved October 14, 2014, from http://www.rsc.org/chemistryworld/News/2009/February/25020901.asp, 2009.
[216] K. Ludlow, D. Bowman, G. Hodge, A Review of Possible Impacts of Nanotechnology on Australia's Regulatory Framework. Retrieved November 14, 2014, from http://www.industry.gov.au/industry/IndustrySectors/nanotechnology/NationalEnablingTechnologiesStrategy/Documents/MonashReport2007.pdf, 2007.
[217] European Commission, Nanosciences and nanotechnologies: An action plan for Europe 2005-2009. Retrieved October 14, 2014, from http://ec.europa.eu/research/industrial_technologies/pdf/nano_action_plan_en.pdf, 2005.
[218] European Commission, Preliminary Opinion Guidance on the Determination of Potential Health Effects of Nanomaterials Used in Medical Devices. Retrieved October 14, 2014, from http://ec.europa.eu/health/scientific_committees/emerging/docs/scenihr_o_045.pdf, 2014.
[219] F. McCaffery, D. McFall, P. Donnelly, F.G. Wilkie, R. Sterritt, in: A software process improvement lifecycle framework for the medical device industry. Engineering of Computer-Based Systems, 2005 ECBS '05 12th IEEE International Conference and Workshops on the 2005, 2005, pp. 273–280.
[220] F. Kevin, J. Blum, Controlling for cybersecurity risks of medical device software, Comm. ACM 56 (2013) 35–37.
[221] C. Lindholm, J.P. Notander, M. Höst, A case study on software risk analysis and planning in medical device development, Softw. Qual. J. 22 (2014) 469–497.
[222] Z. Daw, R. Cleaveland, M. Vetter, Formal verification of software-based medical devices considering medical guidelines, Int. J. Comput. Assist. Radiol. Surg. 9 (2014) 145–153.
[223] M. McHugh, F. McCaffery, V. Casey, Software process improvement to assist medical device software development organisations to comply with the amendments to the medical device directive, Softw. IET 6 (2012) 431–437.
[224] F. McCaffery, V. Casey, M. McHugh, R. O'Connor, J. Pries-Heje, R. Messnarz, How Can Software SMEs Become Medical Device Software SMEs, in: Systems, Software and Service Process Improvement, Springer, Berlin Heidelberg, 2011, pp. 247–258.
[225] Medi SPICE, Introduction. Retrieved October 21, 2014, from http://medispice.ning.com/.
[226] U.S. Food and Drug Administration, Mobile medical applications. Retrieved December 30, 2014, from http://www.fda.gov/MedicalDevices/ProductsandMedicalProcedures/ConnectedHealth/MobileMedicalApplications/ucm255978.htm, 2014.
[227] U.S. Food and Drug Administration, Mobile medical applications—guidance for industry and food and drug administration staff. Retrieved December 30, 2014, from http://www.fda.gov/downloads/MedicalDevices/DeviceRegulationandGuidance/GuidanceDocuments/UCM263366.pdf, 2013.
[228] McKesson, 510(k) Summary McKesson Medical Imaging Company's McKesson Radiology Device, from http://www.accessdata.fda.gov/cdrh_docs/pdf14/K140909.pdf, 2014.

[229] W. Hua-Hsin, Q. Xiaohong, Toward a framework of the process of open innovation: case of Acclarent in the medical device industry, in: 2012 Proceedings of PICMET '12, Technology Management for Emerging Technologies (PICMET), 2012, pp. 3043–3049.

[230] J.B. Pietzsch, M.G. Zanchi, J.H. Linehan, Medical device innovators and the 510(k) Regulatory pathway: implications of a survey-based assessment of industry experience, J. Med. Dev. 6 (2012) 021015.

[231] J.B. Pietzsch, M.G. Zanchi, J.H. Linehan, Medical device innovators and the 510(k) regulatory pathway: implications of a survey-based assessment of industry experience—part 2: medical device ecosystem and policy, J. Med. Dev. 7 (2013) 021003.

[232] D. Zuckerman, P. Brown, A. Das, Lack of publicly available scientific evidence on the safety and effectiveness of implanted medical devices, JAMA Intern. Med. 174 (2014) 1781–1787.

[233] J. Rising, B. Moscovitch, The Food and Drug Administration's Unique Device Identification System: better postmarket data on the safety and effectiveness of medical devices, JAMA Intern. Med. 174 (2014) 1719–1720.

[234] M. Hours, I.È.S. Khati, J. Hamelin, Interference between active implanted medical devices and electromagnetic field emitting devices is rare but real: results of an incidence study in a population of physicians in France, Pacing Clin. Electrophysiol. 37 (2014) 290–296.

[235] Cell phones and electromagnetic interference revisited, Health Devices 35 (2006) 449–456.

[236] E. Occhetta, L. Plebani, M. Bortnik, G. Sacchetti, G. Trevi, Implantable cardioverter defibrillators and cellular telephones: is there any interference? Pacing Clin. Electrophysiol. 22 (1999) 983–989.

[237] J.P. Thaker, M.B. Patel, A.J. Shah, V.V. Liepa, J.D. Brunett, K. Jongnarangsin, et al., Do media players cause interference with pacemakers? Clin. Cardiol. 32 (2009) 653–657.

[238] I. Lavi, G. Malki, R. Kornowski, Medical iPad use in the cardiac catheterization and echo laboratories, Int. J. Cardiovasc. Imaging 30 (2014) 245–252.

[239] K.S. Saini, A. Kaushik, B. Anil, S. Rambabu, Harmonized medical device regulation: need, challenges, and risks of not harmonizing the regulation in Asia, J. Young Pharm. 2 (2010) 101–106.

[240] Organisation for Economic Co-operation and Development, The OECD Report on Regulatory Reform Synthesis. Retrieved January 22, 2015, from http://www.oecd.org/regreform/regulatory-policy/2391768.pdf, 1997.

[241] International Medical Device Regulators Forum, International Medical Device Regulators Forum. Retrieved January 03, 2015, from http://www.imdrf.org/.

[242] International Medical Device Regulators Forum, Meetings. Retrieved January 03, 2015, from http://www.imdrf.org/meetings/meetings.asp.

[243] Asian Harmonization Working Party, About AHWP. Retrieved January 12, 2015, from http://www.ahwp.info/index.php?q=node/7.

[244] Pan American Health Organization, PANDRH. Retrieved January 23, 2015, from http://www.paho.org/hq/index.php?option=com_content&view=category&id=1156&layout=blog&Itemid=1685&lang=en, 2014.

[245] Pan African Harmonization Working Party on Medical Devices and Diagnostics, Pan African Harmonization Working Party on Medical Devices and Diagnostics. Retrieved January 12, 2015, from http://www.pahwp.org/index.html.

[246] Regulatory Affairs Professionsl Society, About RAPS. Retrieved January 12, 2015, from http://www.raps.org/about/.

[247] ASEAN Alliance of Health Supplement Association, About AAHSA. Retrieved January 23, 2015, from http://www.aahsa.org.sg/about/, 2015.

Index

Note: Page numbers followed by *f* indicate figures and *t* indicate tables.